PENGUIN BOOKS

WHY HAVEN'T I LOST WEIGHT YET?

Shane Bilsborough is the author of *The Fat Stripping Diet* and is Australia's best-known personal trainer and lifestyle coach. He is the contributing editor of *Ultra-Fit* magazine. After working as an international model, Shane completed his masters degree in human nutrition and is now a consultant and corporate speaker on weight loss and health for businesses and gyms around Australia.

Johann Bilsborough is a personal training guru with a degree in exercise science. Together, Shane and Johann set up their own personal training and healthy lifestyle management company, B Personal.

For more information, please visit www.bpersonal.com.au

WHY HAVEN'T I LOST WEIGHT YET?

Shane Bilsborough

with

Johann Bilsborough

Penguin Books

Penguin Books

Penguin Group (Australia)
250 Camberwell Road, Camberwell, Victoria 3124, Australia
Penguin Books Ltd
80 Strand, London WC2R 0RL, England
Penguin Group (USA) Inc.
375 Hudson Street, New York, New York 10014, USA
Penguin Books, a division of Pearson Canada
10 Alcorn Avenue, Toronto, Ontario, Canada M4V 3B2
Penguin Books (NZ) Ltd
Cnr Rosedale and Airborne Roads, Albany, Auckland, New Zealand
Penguin Books (South Africa) (Pty) Ltd
24 Sturdee Avenue, Rosebank, Johannesburg 2196, South Africa
Penguin Books India (P) Ltd
11, Community Centre, Panchsheel Park, New Delhi 110 017, India

First published by Penguin Group (Australia), a division of
Pearson Group Pty Ltd, 2004

1 3 5 7 9 10 8 6 4 2

Design by David Altheim © Penguin Group (Australia)
Cover image © photolibrary.com
Author photograph by Tim de Neefe
Typeset in 11/16 pt Minion by Post Pre-press Group, Brisbane, Queensland
Printed and bound in Australia by McPherson's Printing Group, Maryborough, Victoria

National Library of Australia
Cataloguing-in-Publication data:

Bilsborough, Shane.
Why haven't I lost weight yet: you can with the revolutionary Energy Diet.

Includes Index.
ISBN 0 14 300181 7.

1. Reducing diets. I. Bilsborough, Johann. II Title.

613.25

www.penguin.com.au

CONTENTS

INTRODUCTION

'I've been doing all the right things but still can't lose weight!'

So many people are doing what they think are all the right things. You probably eat quite healthily, buy low-fat or 99 per cent fat-free products whenever possible, and do a little exercise. You've even tried all the diets out there! So why can't you get down to your ideal weight?

Why Haven't I Lost Weight Yet? provides a new, easy way of losing weight. It's called the Energy Diet. The Energy Diet is the only diet that looks at the energy density of food. It is this energy density that determines whether we lose weight or gain it. It's that simple: if you want to lose weight, you have to eat 'low energy dense' foods and reduce the 'energy density' of your meals. This book shows you how. By following the

Energy Diet many of our clients at B Personal have lost around 20 kilograms! And they have been able to keep it off for more than 12 months and counting!

The Energy Diet is based on a unique system that will finally allow you to successfully lose weight – the Energy Density Index.

The Energy Density Index, or the EDI, analyses all foods according to the amount of energy they contain. This means the EDI takes into account how much protein, carbohydrate, fat, fibre and water every food contains. All these components contribute to the 'energy of food', and hence the energy it gives you either to use or to store. Knowing the amount and type of energy a food contains is vitally important in your quest to lose weight, as the type of energy (i.e. good or bad) will determine whether you use it as your body's source of fuel or store this energy as fat.

Have you ever wondered how much energy your body actually burns in any given day? How much energy does your body actually need to function? For a typical man this is only 9500 kJ and for a woman 6500 kJ. On average most of us eat somewhere between 11 000 kJ and 14 000 kJ on a typical day. In reality, though, how much food constitutes 9500 kJ and 6500 kJ? If you have tried to lose weight and not succeeded, have a look at the table on the next page, which shows how much food you should be eating. Remember this is the amount of food that your body needs to function.

Woman	Man
1 small bowl of muesli	1 small bowl of muesli
2 pieces of fruit bread	2 pieces of fruit bread
1 apple	1 apple
1 banana	1 banana
1 medium-sized chicken breast	1 large chicken breast
1 carrot	1 carrot
1 small slice of cheese	1 cheese sandwich
	1 small bowl of fruit salad

Shocked? Think about what you ate yesterday, and compare it to this list.

The less energy you eat the more weight you can lose. Using the EDI, you can eat the same *weight* of food you usually do, but by choosing foods that contain lower amounts of energy you will reduce your overall energy intake and therefore reduce your weight.

Now, does this mean that everything discussed in Shane's first two books is obsolete? Certainly not. *The Fat-Stripping Diet* and *7 Days to Strip Fat Forever* combined the latest in human nutrition and weight loss. This new book helps you work through the confusion of all the other diets out there. It looks at why dieting may not have worked for you in the past and shows you that the Energy Diet is fail-safe. It works. Energy Density is the new buzz word when it comes to weight loss and the best thing about it is that it makes sense.

This book is for everyone who wants to shed excess weight, but it is especially for anyone who has tried and previously failed to do so. At last you will find out why before it was so hard to lose weight – and why it is so easy to do so now.

HOW TO USE THIS BOOK

The main idea behind *Why Haven't I Lost Weight Yet?* is to get you to drop those extra kilos you've been trying and trying to lose.

Before starting this program, it is a good idea to have a full medical check-up, particularly if you have any health concerns. Get your heart health, cholesterol and blood pressure checked. Ask for a diabetes check. Explain to the doctor the program you're about to embark upon and take on board any medical suggestions they have.

In order to lose weight most efficiently, we recommend that you start the eating program first (see Chapter 3). It usually takes a little while, about two weeks, to get used to the Energy Density Index and the foods you should be eating, and to get into a stable routine.

How long should you follow the Energy Diet? We hope you can follow this for the rest of your life! The Energy Diet is designed to be simple to use and sustainable in the long term. Of course, there will be days when you lapse or occasionally put the diet aside for a week or so. But if you learn the simple principles of eating low energy foods – rich in fibre and water, low in fat, moderate in carbohydrate and protein – then you will see significant weight loss over a few weeks.

When you feel comfortable with the Energy Diet, you can then start on the Bilsborough Program (see Chapter 7). This is just another aspect of taking charge of your health. With the Bilsborough Program, start at Stage 1 to assess where you are. Then depending on how many steps you take daily, move to Stages 2, 3 or 4. Stay on each stage until you comfortably can manage the next stage. This may be a week to ten days minimum, but is more likely to be three to four weeks. You should aim ultimately to get to Stage 4 or 5. If you are very fit, Stage 5 will suit you, but for many Stage 4 will be the optimum level.

For some of you, you may want to start both the Energy Diet and the Bilsborough Program at the same time. This is fine, but remember that this program is about making small but permanent changes, so allow yourself plenty of time to adapt.

Everyone's response to the diet will be different, depending on how much weight you want to lose. However, we have found that people who follow the Energy Diet in conjunction with the Bilsborough Program on Stages 3 and 4 have lost 10 to 15 kilograms in just over three months.

ENERGY

In this chapter you will learn:

- what energy in food is
- that the amount of food eaten today is greater than ever before
- how to eat right and choose foods for weight loss
- how weight loss will be much easier once you know the energy density of food

Energy for living

The word 'energy' tends to be associated with health and wellbeing. Being energetic is synonymous with having 'get up and go'. Some of us reach for that extra bit of energy in the afternoon or after work to give us the reserves we need to fit more into our lives. Some of us are in dire need of energy just to get through the day, while we watch others around us bursting with energy. Without energy we look and feel tired, worn out and in need of a holiday. Unfortunately, the pressures and rigours of contemporary life mean that we often run out of energy by day's end.

Energy from food

Another way of describing energy is as the energy that food contains. The more food we eat, potentially, but not always, the more energy we eat. Some foods give us the right energy we need to feel fantastic and ready for anything, while energy from other foods is closely linked to its fat content and will make us feel lethargic and not our best.

French fries, for example, will give you plenty of energy but, as most of the energy is in the form of fat, this type of energy may leave you feeling sluggish. We know that energy from fat takes three to four hours to be absorbed, so the energy our bodies get from fat arrives slowly. A bowl of oats with some fresh fruit served in the right amount first thing in the morning, on the other hand, will give you boundless energy without the added weight. We need to find a balance between eating enough of the right foods to put the zip back in our step, and not eating too much food (and hence too much energy) that may lead to fat gain; so portion sizes are important.

The energy in food

Certain food groups have varying amounts of energy, as shown in the table below. There are only four macronutrients that make up our food: fat, carbohydrate, protein and alcohol. Food has other components, such as vitamins, minerals, fibre and water, but only the four macronutrients contribute to the energy of food. Foods containing fat and alcohol give us the most energy per gram, followed by foods containing carbohydrates and protein. (Energy is measured in calories in the USA and kilojoules (kJ) in other countries.)

Macronutrient	Amount	Energy
Fat	(1 gram)	37.8 kJ (9 calories)
Carbohydrate	(1 gram)	16.8 kJ (4 calories)
Protein	(1 gram)	16.8 kJ (4 calories)
Alcohol	(1 gram)	29.4 kJ (7 calories)

The more energy a food has, the more 'energy dense' it is. We refer to the energy found in foods as the 'energy density' of food. Fat and alcohol, for example, are more energy dense than protein or carbohydrates.

In the search for the root of the world's weight-gain

epidemic much time, money and scientific effort are being directed toward establishing the links between weight and fat gains and the energy density of food.

More food than ever before

June, a busy mum, spoke to us after years of unsuccessful weight loss. When we analysed her diet, we saw that she constantly grazed throughout the day. Without realising it, she ate foods that were high in energy density. For example, she ate several pieces of toast with peanut butter for breakfast, chocolate biscuits with her coffee at morning tea, and a tuna salad for lunch. She always nibbled on confectionery and a toasted cheese sandwich when her children came home from school. For dinner she often had a large steak accompanied by small amounts of vegetables, and then ice-cream for dessert. The main skeleton of her eating pattern is okay, with the toast for breakfast, tuna salad for lunch and the steak and some vegetables for dinner, or so it seems. But June actually manages to eat 15 000 kJ worth of energy in a normal day.

Recent evidence shows that we are all consuming more food and hence more energy than ever before. Every time we sit down to eat most of us are overeating and hence consuming extra energy. Whenever our caveman ancestors ate, they tried to eat as much as they could because they never knew when their next meal would come. In today's society we often eat the same way, although food has never before been so over-abundant.

The next time you sit down with friends, watch how the

people around you eat. The signal that people have finished eating is usually given by comments of 'I couldn't possibly fit another thing in', or sighs of 'I'm full'.

The amounts of food we consume daily are massive, and much more than our bodies are equipped to metabolise in a given day. This has seen people grow larger in the Western world, especially in the USA, the UK and Australia. This is despite the number of low-fat products on the market, the millions of people worldwide who have been reducing their cabohydrate intake for over 10 years, and the use of other fad methods of dieting that don't control the energy density of food.

More energy than we can use

An average man eats 11 500 kJ and an average woman eats 8000 kJ daily. For those who eat more than average there are dire health consequences. Data suggests that in the USA people spend $220 billion on restaurants and fast food annually and about $40 billion each year on some form of weight loss therapy.

In the USA 97.1 million people are overweight or obese, which is 65 per cent of the population. This is five times the actual population of Australia. For children the value is about 10 per cent and growing at a massive rate. But the phenomenon of large weight gain is not confined to the USA. The British population is 48 per cent overweight or obese, and this is expected to come close to 60 per cent by 2006. Germany has an overweight/obese population of 57 per cent and this is predicted to grow to 71 per cent by 2006, while Spain and the Netherlands have levels of 69 per cent and are expected to reach 80 per cent by 2006. Some 60 per cent of Australians are overweight, 25 to 30 per cent are obese. Obesity in Australia was 8 per cent for women and 9.3 per cent for men back in 1980. In 2002 these levels rose to 21.8 per cent for women and 19.1 per cent for men.

This huge rise in weight gain (especially on the tummy area) is paralleled by the increase in cases of diabetes around the world. A former client of ours, Ron, demonstrates how over-eating can lead to diabetes. Ron never ate breakfast, but ate a huge lunch, sometimes sandwiches or pies but always hot chips, and an even larger dinner with a serving of fries and often ice-cream, cakes, biscuits and chocolate to follow. His most intriguing comment was, 'But I don't eat a lot of sugar!', mistakenly thinking diabetes is brought about by eating too much sugar. If you, like Ron, are eating large meals, and energy-rich snacks then you could unknowingly be on the slow journey towards diabetes. In 1985 worldwide estimates were 30 million cases of late-onset diabetes caused by weight gain. This grew to 135 million by 1995, and is expected to reach 300 to 500 million by 2025. This means by that year about 10 per cent of the world's population will have weight-gain-associated diabetes.

In 2025 about 75–90 per cent of the population in most countries will be overweight or obese. This is a time when Western diseases will strike at our children as well as us. This is what needs to be seriously considered.

Weight gain has everything to do with the energy density of the food we eat, and very little else. If you have been trying for years to lose weight, and are confused by the numerous fads on the market, then understanding energy density is the first step.

What is energy density?

The term 'energy density' is used to describe the amount of energy that food contains, as we saw on page 9. The energy density of a food depends on the amount of fat, carbohydrates and protein found in that food. The more of these macro-nutrients, the greater the energy density level. Alcohol too contains energy. Fibre and water also have an impact on the energy density of the food we eat.

Let's use some practical examples to explain energy density and how it can be relevant to weight loss.

FOOD (100 grams)	WATER (grams)	FAT (grams)	CARBOHYDRATE/ PROTEIN (grams)	FIBRE (grams)	ENERGY DENSITY (kJ)
broccoli	88.7	0.3	5.3	4.1	137
cheese	41.4	32.4	20.4	0	1570
chocolate	1.5	32.4	61.6 (55.4 g carbs + 6.2 g protein)	0.5	2200

Very simply, foods that are low in fat, carbohydrates and protein and high in fibre and water are low energy dense foods. Foods that are low in fibre and water and high in fat, carbohydrates and protein are high energy dense foods. As the above table shows, broccoli contains large amounts of water and fibre, low amounts of fat, carbohydrates and proteins and, above all, has only 137 kJ of energy in a 100 gram serving. In terms of energy density, broccoli is considered a low energy dense food. As you will see in Chapter 3, the idea is to consume low energy density foods as much as possible to aid the reduction of body fat and hence weight.

To start with, a 100 gram slice of cheese is much smaller than a 100 gram serving of broccoli, and contains less water. As we will see later the more water a food contains the less energy dense it is, and hence the more beneficial it is for weight regulation. Although cheese has larger amounts of protein (20.4 grams compared to 0.4 grams), it has 108 times the amount of fat (32.4 grams of fat to 0.3 grams), and over 11 times the energy density (1570 kJ compared to 137 kJ). The other feature of cheese is that it contains absolutely no fibre.

The more fat a food contains, the more energy it contains; and of course the lower the amount of fat in the food, the lower the energy density of the food. The main difference between cheese and broccoli is the fat content, and this accounts for the massive difference in the energy of the two foods. Although in the past we have focused mainly on fat, this book gives us the room to expand further the concept of energy and how it is so strongly linked to weight gain or loss. However, we must still emphasise that the amount of fat we consume is still a large part of weight gain.

As the table on the previous page clearly shows, chocolate contains essentially no water, large amounts of fat and large amounts of carbohydrates (primarily in the form of sugar: 55.4 grams) and smaller amounts of protein (6.2 grams). Chocolate has virtually no fibre and has a whopping energy density of 2200 kJ. The difference between chocolate and cheese is remarkable in that both have similar amounts of fat (32.4 grams each), but 100 grams of chocolate has three times as much energy from carbohydrate/protein.

A 100 gram block of chocolate is extremely high in energy density, and if you ate a 250 gram block of chocolate by yourself, your energy density intake would increase to 5375 kJ. Keep in mind that an average man eats 11 500 kJ daily and an average woman eats 8000 kJ daily. This shows that in one sitting it is possible to consume nearly 70 per cent of your day's energy from a large block of chocolate!

The energy of this chocolate comes from 32.4 grams of fat and 55.4 grams of sugar. The sugar is absorbed from the small intestine quite quickly and then stored in the liver and muscles as glycogen. The energy released from the sugar is a short burst lasting between 30 minutes and one hour, which is why you often experience a high or a burst of energy immediately after eating some chocolate. It takes fat about three hours to be made into a transportable form and then absorbed into the circulation, so this means our 32.4 grams of fat takes around five hours to be stored around the body as fat.

Another characteristic chocolate and cheese have in common is their fibre content. Chocolate contains very little fibre. Cheese contains none at all. Fibre is what makes us feel full, and so the reason we can consume plenty of chocolate and cheese before we feel full is their lack of fibre.

Energy calculations

To calculate the energy density of food, multiply the macronutrient content by the amount of energy in 1 gram of that macronutrient (using the table on page 9). This calculation shows that fat contributes 1225 kJ of energy to both cheese and chocolate. For cheese this is 78 per cent of the total energy and for chocolate this is 54 per cent. The contribution of carbohydrates and protein to cheese and chocolate is 22 per cent and 46 per cent respectively.

	Cheese	Chocolate
Fat (grams)	32.4	32.4
Energy from fat (kJ)	32.4 × 37.8 = 1225 kJ	32.4 × 37.8 = 1225 kJ
Carbohydrate/protein (grams)	20.4	61.6
Energy from carbohydrate/ protein (kJ)	20.4 × 16.8 = 343 kJ	61.6 × 16.8 =1035 kJ
Total energy	1225 + 343 ~1570 kJ	1225 + 1035 ~2260 kJ

The Energy Density Index

We have unearthed something revolutionary and scientifically based that actually has a huge amount to do with weight loss – the Energy Density Index. Let's clarify once and for all the facts about weight loss.

- It's the energy content of the food that is extremely important, above all other factors.
- It is the energy density of food, not the GI nor the carbohydrate content or people's blood type (see Chapter 2), that seems to be linked with weight gain. And this is supported by numerous medical journals.
- It is the energy density of food that science has clearly linked to weight gain and obesity, above and beyond anything else.
- It is the energy density of food – not blood types, dirty livers, carbohydrate addiction or Syndrome X, Y or Z – that is the topic of concern at international obesity conferences.

These are the facts and this book is based solely on these scientifically supported facts.

The Energy Density Index turns out to be the real solution to weight loss. We will show you how the EDI can be used as a tool in weight loss in almost every aspect of life, whether this be eating fast food, eating out at a restaurant, deciding which foods to choose or even having a drink on Friday night. We will also demonstrate how the EDI affects exercise.

If we turn our attention back to page 8, we discussed the concept of having more energy. The EDI will allow you to get the right type of energy for vitality, without consuming the type of energy that leads to weight gain. Trialling the EDI with our large client base at B Personal, we have achieved results that are nothing short of sensational.

Top 10 points to remember about energy
1 All food contains energy.
2 Fat contains 2.25 times more energy per gram than carbohydrates or protein.
3 Excess energy usually gets stored as fat.
4 Larger portion sizes of food contain larger amounts of energy.
5 A low-fat product should contain less energy than its full-fat equivalent.
6 By reducing fat consumption and increasing fibre consumption we can reduce the amount of energy we eat.
7 A low-carb diet substitutes fat for carbohydrate and can therefore increase energy intake.
8 Energy is measured in kilojoules.
9 Alcohol can significantly contribute to energy storage.
10 Most diets fail because they don't factor in energy.

Summary

This is the first book to address the issue of energy intake and the relationship between weight gain and the energy of foods. While the blame for why we gain fat and weight has shifted around all sorts of theories, there is a mass of medical evidence showing that it is now essentially the energy density of food that is making us larger by the minute. It is the energy density of food that is the key reason for not losing weight, despite doing all the right things.

If you are eating more low-fat foods, going for the occasional walk, and you've even switched to drinking red wine, but have not considered the amount of energy your food contains, then all these small changes are useless as far as weight loss is concerned and may only remove a droplet of fat from a vast ocean of extra kilos!

WHY PEOPLE STILL AREN'T LOSING WEIGHT

In this chapter you will learn:

- why eating low-fat foods does not always lead to weight loss
- why a low-carbohydrate diet is not the answer
- what the Glycemic Index is and why it doesn't work for weight loss
- why low-fat diets don't always work
- that without controlling your daily energy intake you will inevitably consume more energy than your body needs

Top 10 reasons why people don't lose weight

1 People never stick to diets.
2 People often eat chocolate/sweets even when they're dieting.
3 People believe they are eating low-fat but in reality they are only eating *lower*-fat foods.
4 People eat too much food.
5 Fad diets don't work.
6 People are not active during a typical day.
7 People eat off larger plates, making large meals look small.
8 People eat too quickly.
9 People don't like to deprive themselves of food.
10 People tend to eat until they are full.

The low-fat diet

Low-fat foods and low-fat diets have been around for decades now. At some time we've all tried to eat less fat, so why aren't we getting any thinner?

Margaret has attempted to lose weight by following what she thought was a low-fat diet. She weighed 80 kg when she started and wanted to get down to 65 kg for a wedding she had coming up in six months. What did she do? She essentially bought and ate low-fat foods! But thinking she could eat as much low-fat food as she liked – because it was low-fat – she ended up eating even more food than before. She would eat a whole packet of low-fat biscuits, lots of low-fat yoghurt (she never bothered to read the labels and choose a low fat/low sugar yoghurt). She never once ate less food.

Her weight didn't change for the first month and then in the first week of the second month she gained a kilogram. Her fat intake was reduced from 123 grams to 88 grams of fat per day, but her engery intake for the day was still 9876 kJ, too much to offset any weight loss. We constantly have people emailing us saying that they are following low-fat diets but are not losing weight. How can this be? On further investigation we found that a staggering 76 per cent of people emailing us with their daily eating plans are eating 83 grams of fat (women) and 87 grams of fat (men) or more per day. This is much more fat than the body can burn off in one day! We found that 84 per cent of women and 87 per cent of men who claimed they couldn't lose weight had energy intakes greater than 8500 kJ and 12 200 kJ respectively.

One of the biggest problems for low-fat dieters seems to be that they eat well for most of the day, then at some point eat something that compromises their diet. But when you don't know the energy density of food, you can't control your energy intake. A close analysis of the food consumed reveals that for most of the day the dieter eats well until they go out for dinner, get some takeaway or eat someone else's cooking. When you don't control food preparation, it is difficult to know what's in it and how much energy it contains.

Another area where a diet low in fat fails is when people eat well for four days of the week and then eat whatever comes their way for the other three days. Once again this is not conducive to weight loss. All the good work of the first four days is lost on the weekend.

So while our clients think they are eating a low-fat diet and therefore should be losing weight, their energy intake needs to be considered. The first point to understand is that this diet is simply too high in energy to promote any weight loss. Remember that foods that are very high in energy are often small and unassuming. The muffin and chocolate biscuits are clear examples of this.

Another failing of a low-fat diet is that people simply reduce their fat intake rather than actually eat foods that are low in energy. The real effect of this isn't fat loss but a slow fat gain. This means that although people think their diet is low in fat (by eating low-fat or 99 per cent fat-free foods), it is actually still relatively high in fat and energy – because they are concentrating on the fat content of foods rather than the energy density.

People who understand that a reduction in fat also means a reduction in the energy they eat can lose weight successfully and keep it off in the long term. Our database shows nearly 1000 people lost more than 20 kilograms by following a low-energy diet. After all, this is the whole aim of a diet lower in fat – to lower energy.

Are low-fat foods low in energy?
Plenty of people think that as long as they are eating low-fat foods they can eat as much food as they want. This is part of the problem! Just because you're eating low-fat food doesn't mean that you can eat more food than ever before.

We have discovered some earth-shattering scientific relationships that will make us all think harder about what we eat. In one study (soon to be published) we researched whether low-fat foods are lower in actual energy than their full-fat counterparts. Remember, the reason we want to reduce fat is to reduce energy, not consume more energy from sugar.

We collected over 400 foods that had a full-fat product and a low-fat product from the same manufacturers. This way we were able to analyse what the manufacturing company meant by low-fat, lite or 97 per cent fat-free. For example, company X may have had a full-cream ice-cream and a 97 per cent fat-free ice-cream. Did the low-fat ice-cream have lower energy than the full-fat product, or did the manufacturer just take out the fat and replace it with sugar?

In sweet foods, we discovered that the energy in a low-fat product is virtually no different from the energy in a full-fat product. Low-fat sweet products have only 3 per cent lower energy than their high-fat counterparts. Low-fat savoury products, however (as shown in the table opposite), were much lower in fat than full-fat savoury products. The difference between a full-fat savoury product and a low-fat one is 35 per cent or about 400 kJ (95 calories).

So, while aiming for low-fat products you may inadvertently have been eating energy dense foods that prevented you from losing weight. Does this mean then that all low-fat foods are useless and we may as well eat the full-fat versions? Certainly not. Because fat has 2¼ times more energy than protein or carbohydrate, cutting down on fat means cutting down on energy. This is simple mathematics: the less fat you eat, the less energy you eat. To buy the best 'weight-loss' food, you should check the fat as well as the sugar content, as some low-fat foods may still be high in energy.

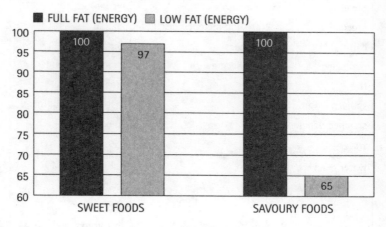

(from Bilsborough, Cameron-Smith & Crowe, 2002 unpublished data)

Just can't stop eating!

Scientists call the great taste sensation that fat has 'palatability'. When we eat we are governed by taste more often than not. We like food that tastes good, and if we were to give you a choice between a carrot and a piece of chocolate, we have absolutely no doubt that the chocolate would win every time. If we cast our minds back to when we were children we may at some time have had trouble eating the vegetables on our plate, such as brussels sprouts, because we didn't like the taste. But we abandoned the greens and dived into the ice-cream. That's palatability in action.

FOOD Low palatability	FOOD Moderate palatability	FOOD High palatability
bread	bananas	alcohol
broccoli	dry unsweetened biscuits	cheese
carrots	oranges	chocolate
pumpkin	salad sandwich	chocolate biscuits
rice		cream cakes
spinach		fast food hamburgers
steamed vegetables		french fries
water		ice-cream
water crackers		lollies
		pastries
		pies
		soft drinks

Studies have repeatedly shown that high palatability foods are those which contain the most energy and fat. In fact, there is a strong relationship between energy density and palatability.

The signals to the brain for us to stop eating are triggered by certain foods, and delayed by other foods. Foods containing water promote satiation by stimulating receptors in the stomach, which communicate with the brain. It is thought that foods containing fat actually delay the sensation of fullness. That is, when consuming a fatty meal, the signal that goes to the brain to say 'I'm full' is put on hold. This is clearly shown by comparing the fat in cheese to a cooked potato (with no added oil, butter or sour cream). The potato (high water and fibre content, low in fat) would be much more filling than cheese (low in water, low in fibre and high in fat). The potato sets off a trigger in the brain to stop you eating more food, but not so after the same amount of cheese. This causes a huge practical problem in our quest for short- and long-term weight loss. Firstly, after the potato (100 grams) you would finish eating and feel quite full, having eaten 350 kJ of energy and 0 grams of fat. After 100 grams of cheese, the brain still has not recognised that you've eaten enough, so you are more inclined to have another 100 grams or more, before feeling full.

This results in 200 grams of cheese, 65 grams of fat and a whopping 3100 kJ of energy. (Again, keep in mind that an average man eats 11 500 kJ and a woman eats 8000 kJ daily.) In a single sitting it is possible to consume three times as much energy eating foods that contain fat, compared to carbohydrate or protein. Ask yourself why it is that you can eat large amounts of fast food, restaurant food, ice-cream, chocolate, cheese, bacon and fatty foods – and not so many brussel sprouts. You need to eat more before the body says enough is enough. Anyone searching for a solution to weight loss is certainly not going to lose weight consuming foods in this category.

Many pharmaceutical drugs are being developed focusing

on this part of our appetite. These drugs try to get the brain to trigger the process of 'fullness' after consuming very little food.

Food portion sizes

Our quest to lose weight permanently has been grossly challenged in the past because there was no way we could control the energy of our food and consequently the amount of energy we ate. The tools we used failed us because all rules go out the window when you don't understand the energy content of food.

Energy-dense food is consumed in the greatest amounts in Western society. One study in the *American Journal of Clinical Nutrition* (December 2002) investigated how we eat when we are presented with four different portion sizes of macaroni and cheese: 500 grams, 625 grams, 750 grams and 1000 grams. When people were asked to choose their own meal sizes, most chose the biggest portion size and ate more food – even though they weren't hungry. It's part of our mentality to select the biggest option and to not waste it. In today's society, it is very common to reach for the large muffin, a main size dish, and go back for seconds, even while we are on a diet, or even when we are not hungry. The most bizarre thing is that few of us even notice we are doing it!

One significant way to avoid weight gain is to understand portion sizes. To control the energy density of the food we eat, we need to eat smaller portions of high energy dense foods and larger portions of low energy dense foods. Portion sizes of our meals have increased by a staggering amount in recent times and, with energy dense foods, this has meant that the energy of each of our meals has also skyrocketed. This has not been an overnight change, but rather a gradual shift over a period of 20 to 30 years. Recent scientific evidence shows that when we sit down to eat a meal or even a simple snack, the amount of food we are consuming grossly exceeds what health experts recommend. In the *American Journal of Public Health* (March 2002), Dr Lisa Young reported just how much food we're really eating. For example, the differences in portion sizes of ready-to-eat prepared foods and standard US Department of Agriculture [USDA] and US Food and Drug Administration [FDA] portion sizes show that:

- today's cookie sizes exceed a standard cookie size by over 700%
- muffins exceed a standard size muffin by 333%
- hamburgers are 112% bigger
- french fries portions are 168% larger
- bagels are 195% larger
- steaks are 224% bigger
- a glass of beer is between 28–93% greater than recommended
- a slice of pizza is 42% larger
- a serving of pasta is 190–480% larger
- soft drinks are between 35%–103% greater than recommended serves.

If you have had trouble losing weight in the past, how do your meal sizes stack up to the ones reported in the study? Are you unknowingly purchasing the cake-size muffin when in reality the small one is all you really feel like? Have you ever got halfway through the muffin, and thought, 'I'm so full', but continued to finish the whole thing anyway? Are you going to a restaurant that serves steak the size of half a cow, when your body only needs the energy from a hand-sized piece of meat? Have you ever bought 'four for the price of one' food items like doughnuts, and eaten them not because you needed them or the energy they contained, but because you found a food bargain and overate because you could?

As these statistics show, we are getting extremely great value for money, but certainly not from a weight loss or health perspective. As our food portion sizes increase, we consume more energy. This is an unfortunate fact. A standard 200 gram piece of steak contains 1600 kJ of energy. A steak 224 per cent greater in portion size contains 3600 kJ, or 2000 extra kilojoules that a person just doesn't need. A standard-sized muffin nets you 900 kJ, while a muffin 333 per cent larger boosts this to about 2600 kJ. Are your choices of food upsizing your waistline even though most of the time you do the right things in order to lose weight?

The low-carbohydrate diet

Chris went on a low-carbohydrate diet for 12 weeks. She initially lost about 4 kg eating essentially meat and fats, and no carbohydrates. She even cut down on her fruit and vegetables, as she found out that they also contained carbohydrates. She struggled to maintain this diet, always feeling tired and run-down. The final straw for Chris was when her hair started to thin, and her nails became brittle, and would break easily. What was happening to Chris was that her body was taking the protein she ate, and rather than use her protein for growth and repair, it was broken down and used as a carbohydrate. This explains her hair and nail horror story. After plateauing with her initial weight loss (which was undoubtedly water and muscle loss), her weight started to creep back on, and she ended up 4 kg heavier than when she started the diet.

In worldwide conferences where people are invited to submit plans, evidence or solutions to the obesity epidemic, few front up with any research on low-carbohydrate diets as a long-term weight-loss solution. There have been more diet books on low-carbohydrate diets sold worldwide than any other form of diet, yet from 1992 to 2002 cases of overweight and obesity increased at a much greater rate than between 1982 and 1992.

Drawing simple conclusions like this may be a little flippant, but there is some truth in them. The low-carbohydrate guide-lines suggest that by leaving out carbohydrate foods weight gain and obesity problems are solved. When we speak at corporate and fitness conferences we are often told that some people don't even eat fruit as they believe that fruit (a carbohydrate) can lead to weight gain. Do the advocates of low-carbohydrate diets sug-gest that you can eat as much cheese, chocolate, alcohol, fast food and protein as you like as long as you don't eat pasta, bread or rice? Yes, this is unfortunately the message, and although low-carbohydrate diets indirectly are supposed to provide lower amounts of energy, the over-consumption of fat increases the amount of energy we eat.

We receive a multitude of emails each week at B Personal from people asking why they are not losing weight on a low-carbohydrate/high-protein diet despite all the hype that these types of diets come with.

These diets are a shocking excuse to eat foods that most of us consider to be synonymous with weight gain rather than loss. Foods such as bacon, cheese, fat on meat and oils are very commonly consumed in low-carbohydrate diets. If you have tried and failed to lose weight on a low-carbohydrate diet, this could be why.

There may be some days of low energy on a low-carbohydrate diet, but continual consumption of high-fat foods, cheese, chocolate and alcohol makes up for these low-energy days. Both the low-fat diet and the low-carbohydrate diet show how people may be following a particular diet – in the hope of weight loss – but are still consuming more energy than they need.

The Syndrome X diet

What about Syndrome X, which in scientific terms is a real disease? It is a name used to group together diabetes, overweight or obesity, high cholesterol and high blood pressure. Cutting down your carbohydrates (as is often suggested in such cases), however, is not the cure for Syndrome X, and clinical studies have shown that cutting down carbohydrates can worsen diabetes, cholesterol and blood pressure. In fact, we now know some diabetic people can safely eat the same amount of sugar as non-diabetic people!

There are some claims that with Syndrome X there is a chemical imbalance that makes people store fat. To suggest that all people who gain weight have the same chemical imbalance and store weight more easily because of this, rather than due to the fact that they eat plenty of food and don't exercise, is a cop-out. Yes, we all have a genetic predisposition to gain weight, and no one living today is exempt: if we all ate too much we would ultimately gain weight and develop associated diseases. Many people still believe that good quality carbohydrates will make them fat, or give them diabetes and heart disease, and shorten their life span. This is just not the case. As with other eating plans, it is the total energy consumption that is of vital importance, yet this doesn't rate a mention.

The 'eat right for your blood type' diet

This is another example of a diet that doesn't control the energy density of food. Sonia followed the blood type diet, which suggests that people eat certain foods according to their specific blood type. Sonia's blood type is type O, so it has been suggested that she eat plenty of meat and protein, little carbohydrate and avoid dairy products. Sonia's husband Peter also followed the foods that his blood type (type AB) suggest:

high carbohydrates, plenty of fruit and vegetables, low fat and lower protein. It was recommended not to consume meat, dairy products and animal fats. Neither Sonia or Peter had lost any weight in 15 weeks on the diet and so they contacted us to ask why? The simple answer was that they were both consuming much more energy than their bodies were able to metabolise in a day, eating about 8678 kJ and 12 369 kJ for Sonia and Peter respectively. Both were also inactive!

Eating according to your blood type once again puts no restriction on the relative amount of energy you can consume. More importantly, food cannot affect your blood type, which is determined by your genes. Followers of this diet confuse their blood type with what is actually *in* the blood, such as minerals, proteins, hormones and vitamins. You can change what's in your blood but you cannot change your blood type, and no medical evidence exists to support such a claim. At obesity conferences blood types are never mentioned as a factor in weight loss.

The Glycemic Index (GI) diet

One diet that has gained a lot of momentum in the last few years, particularly in Australia, is based on the Glycemic Index or GI. The most important question that we get asked is what the Glycemic Index has to do with weight loss. Basically – nothing.

Gale decided to lose weight by following her version of the GI diet. She basically cut back on carbohydrates but ate as much fat and protein as she liked. Her weight changed very little on this diet. Foods such as cheese with a GI of '0' give people the false impression that they can be eaten in volume. Gale believed she could eat as much cheese and chocolate as she liked, as these foods didn't contain large amounts of carbohydrates or were low-moderate GI foods. She even saw a chocolate spread, which contains massive amounts of fat and sugar, advertised on TV as a low GI food. No wonder she couldn't lose weight.

The Glycemic Index is a measurement (from 1 to 100) of how much glucose a carbohydrate food produces in the bloodstream, two hours after it has been eaten. It is thought that the insulin response to glucose is instrumental in weight loss. Therefore if a digested food produces a low level of glucose in the blood stream, the better the chances of weight loss. All foods are compared to the value of 100, which is that of glucose. As an example, if glucose releases 100 units of glucose, then red kidney beans and lentils release only 27 and 26 units respectively. The goal of following the GI way of eating is to eat low GI foods, and avoid foods that have a high GI (such as potatoes, which have a GI of 85).

This all sounds quite simple – except there are some major problems. There is absolutely no evidence to date to suggest that eating low GI foods alone will result in long-term weight loss, because the Glycemic Index does not take into account the amount of energy in food. In the following table you will be able to see that eating a majority of foods with a low energy correlates much better to weight loss than eating just low GI foods.

Watermelon contains carbohydrates (in the form of fruit sugars), which when broken down produce glucose in our bloodstream. The GI measures how much glucose is present in the bloodstream in the two hours after a food like watermelon has been eaten. The GI of watermelon is 72. However, a 100 gram piece of watermelon contains a mere 138 kJ of energy. This means a food such as watermelon is extremely low in energy, high in fibre and water, and low in fat. Health professionals around the world have been encouraging people to eat these kinds of foods for years. There is nothing unhealthy about watermelon, yet many people have told us they have cut tropical fruits such as watermelon from their diets and the diets of their children. Why? Because the Glycemic Index says to stay away from foods with a high GI, they say. On the GI diet people are advised to eat low to moderate GI foods.

FOOD (100 grams)	GI	FAT (grams)	ENERGY (kJ)
watermelon	72	0	138
oats (cooked)	66	0	199
potato	85	0	256
banana	52	0	377
cheese	0	32	1570
chocolate	32	33	2200

Using the GI, we learn that watermelon is a high GI food, but cheese and chocolate have low and moderate GIs! The confusion continues. A GI value of 66 suggests that oats are a 'medium' GI food, and many people staring at a number of 66 may confuse this with being a food they should avoid. Potatoes are a further example of the inconsistency of a GI-based diet. The GI of potato is 85, yet the energy in a 100 gram serving is only 256 kJ and the fat content is 0. (How many people, though, add cream, cheese or butter to their mashed potatoes? How many people use oil when cooking potatoes? Potatoes alone are harmless, but how we cook them really changes their energy content.)

Cheese is often consumed in quantities on GI diets as it has a GI of about 0. Yet its kilojoule content of 1570 kJ suggests that the energy it contains is too high for it to be considered to be a healthy food that can be consumed at any time. What contributes to cheese's high energy density is the 32 grams of fat per 100 gram serving. Adding fat to a meal lowers the GI, but the GI does not promote large amounts of fat.

The GI – a useful weight-loss tool?
Leading weight-loss scientist, Dr F Xavier Pi-Sunyer, was asked to monitor and assess the Glycemic Index over the last 20 years. His findings were reported in 'Glycemic Index and Disease' in the *American Journal of Clinical Nutrition* (2002).

> Because of the many uncertainties regarding the validity of the GI for determining what foods are 'good' or 'bad' for one's health, I believe it would be a mistake to initiate a public health campaign stating that certain widely consumed carbohydrates should be avoided . . . The prevention of type 2 diabetes is a critical public health priority, given that the prevalence of diabetes in the US population has increased from 8.9 per cent to 12.3 per cent in 11 years, and continues to increase. The rate of obesity, a primary predictor of diabetes, is skyrocketing. As a matter of public health, the message is clear: **decrease total energy intakes and increase physical activity.** To decrease the incidence of cardiovascular disease, lifestyle changes and low saturated fat intakes are recommended. These are recommendations that we can all agree on.

So, our energy intake is at the root of the obesity epidemic, and a reduction in kilojoules is what we must focus on, rather than using an unproven weight-loss tool such as the GI.

There are some very sound and practical uses for the GI. If you have diabetes then eating foods with a low to moderate GI value, such as lentils, red kidney beans, mixed grain breads, or fruits such as apples and oranges may help with the greatest challenge to diabetics – keeping blood glucose levels down (although the GI is not recognised by the American Diabetic Association).

But how can the Glycemic Index help with weight loss? Does the medical evidence suggest that if a person eats all low GI foods that they will lose weight?

To date there is no good long-term evidence that a low GI diet leads to weight loss. This is a medical fact.

One study, see the *American Journal of Clinical Nutrition* (by Bente Kiens and Erik Richer, 1996), observed people eating as much food as they wanted over 30 days, from either low-GI foods or high-GI foods. Weight loss in either group was not significant between those who ate either a high or low GI diet. A second two-week study also found no differences in weight loss.

Although foods in Australia have been labelled with their GI values, the acceptance of GI across the world is not uniform. (Foods in Australia are labelled according to their Glycemic Index, but this lead has not been followed by the USA or the UK.) Many scientists are appalled by the willingness to accept and use the GI for weight loss when the evidence of its true effects is as yet not conclusive. Recently advocates of the GI have refined their data to develop the GL – Glycemic Load – which may be a better tool than the GI. The American Diabetes Association, the American Dietetic Association, and the American Heart Association do not recognise the GI as a tool in the treatment of disease, never mind weight loss. These three influential health institutions recognise that there are many inconsistencies in the use of the GI as a weight-loss tool.

The exercise diet

Jenny went on an exercise diet and was transformed from *Jenny the couch dweller* to *Jenny the fitness guru*. Going from doing nothing Jenny began power-walking, went to the gym three times a week, and filled her pantry with healthy food and drinks. She was super motivated. Initially her weight dropped from 77 kg to 68 kg. This was wonderful for Jenny and really does typify the power of physical activity for weight loss. Reaching her goal weight Jenny naively believed that she had reached the finish line with her eating and exercising. So she stopped exercising and resumed her normal eating. If you stop, like Jenny did, and revert back to your previous inactive lifestyle, your weight will go straight back on. Jenny ended up back at 77 kg

The problem with most exercise diets is that they involve a full-on physical commitment to drop the necessary weight. It is difficult to sustain a high-exercise diet, so if you don't change your eating patterns, you can expect the weight will pile back on once you stop exercising.

However, if we're considering some form of mild exercise to combine with the diets described earlier, we have an even more significant problem. Apart from the fact that the energy intake from these diets is much greater than it should be – and therefore inhibits weight loss – recent studies have revealed an alarming drop in the amount we move each day. Here we're not talking about physical activity such as running or walking, we mean the amount of time we spend on our feet – rather than sitting at a desk or in front of the television. *The amount of energy the average person expends each day is about equivalent to the energy that's contained in an apple.* So even if you think you're dieting correctly, if you're not moving around much then your weight loss will be minimal. More importantly, if you're exercising three times a week but not losing weight, it means that you're still not expending more energy than you're consuming. See Chapter 8 for the best exercise for permanent weight loss.

Summary

Very few diets help us to eat less energy than our body burns. In clinical trials, weight loss is achieved quite comfortably but when people resume a Western lifestyle the weight can be regained in less than six months. The key to weight loss is in reducing the energy you consume and increasing the energy you expend.

THE ENERGY DIET

In this chapter you will learn:

- to use the Energy Density Index (EDI) to determine how much energy food contains
- low EDI foods promote weight loss
- high EDI foods promote weight gain
- the EDI is the only weight-loss tool you need
- all EDI values are approximates only

A new way of counting calories

The best model of weight management is one that takes into account fat, carbohydrates, protein and hence the energy of food. Strangely no model of weight loss has done this until now. What if we could develop a weight-loss tool that puts all foods on an equal playing field, giving you a no-nonsense guide to choosing lower energy foods no matter what the food contains? What if that tool also enabled astounding results with weight loss? With the help, guidance and encouragement of some of the world's best scientists in obesity, weight control, exercise metabolism and mathematics, we have come up with such a tool: The Energy Density Index.

Evidence does exist to show that eating foods that are low in energy density can lead not only to very significant weight loss, but also to reductions in cholesterol, blood pressure, insulin resistance and the risk of diabetes. In every study that significantly reduced the energy density of people's diets, weight loss eventuated. This is the most convincing aspect of the Energy Density Index.

How can we choose foods that are lower in energy?

There are several factors you need to consider in order to choose low energy density foods. By understanding why you are selecting a particular food you are more empowered to take control of your weight than if you were simply to follow a diet without any real understanding of how it works.

Water

There is a very strong relationship between water and energy density and hence water-containing foods and weight loss. This important relationship means that the more water-containing foods you consume the less energy you will consume. This is clearly demonstrated earlier when evaluating 100 grams of broccoli (see page 13). Like broccoli, almost all fruit and vegetables contain about 90 per cent of their weight as water. Water-containing foods have a greater tendency to fill you up, as opposed to foods that contain little water, such as cheese and chocolate. Think of a bowl of clear broth or soup. You may only consume a small amount but the liquid nature of the food promotes a filling effect. Foods with a high water content are listed on the following page, and these foods contain little carbohydrate, protein and energy.

In 1998 Dr Barbara Rolls, a prominent figure in energy density research, looked at how consuming a larger volume of water affects the energy a person consumed. In this study men were given a milk-based drink at approximately 30 minutes before lunch. It was shown that after drinking 600 ml of liquid before lunch, the amount of food a person eats can be cut by 17.6 per cent, which may demonstrate the importance of consuming water/liquid/soup-based foods prior to lunch to reduce the energy density of food.

One reason for this decreased energy intake when volumes of food are consumed has to do with receptors found in our stomach. These pressure sensors are touched or stimulated by the water that soup contains, or the water from a fruit salad, for example. When these receptors are stimulated they trigger a signal to the brain to stop eating. The large consumption of water-based foods (such as rice noodle soups) may be one reason why Asian people manage to eat smaller amounts of food than Westerners, stay leaner and are less likely to put on weight. Other data show that when the majority of foods consumed during the day contain more water, the amount of energy eaten is significantly reduced, sometimes by as much as 40 per cent.

It is important then to consume plenty of fruit, vegetables and vegetable-based dishes and to use more water in foods, such as by adding an extra cup of water to a pasta sauce or casserole (do this close to serving time to cut down on evaporation). The main thing is to ensure that your meals have a greater than normal water content to increase feelings of fullness and to lower energy density.

Top 10 water-containing meals
1 Vegetable soup or any water-based soup
2 Rice noodles/rice noodle soups
3 Vegetable lasagne
4 Vegetable risotto
5 Pasta with legumes such as cannellini beans
6 Pasta with vegetables such as asparagus/zucchini
7 Couscous with vegetables
8 Mixed bean salad (red kidney beans, chickpeas, cannellini beans, green beans)

9 Salad sandwich (tomato, lettuce, cucumber, carrot in wholemeal bread)

10 Fruit salad

Fibre

The role of fibre is essential to weight loss and has an interesting role to play in the energy density of food. Our caveman ancestors ate between 77 and 120 grams of fibre each day. Today's estimates are 15 grams per day in the USA and 20 grams in Australia. In countries where 'overweightness' is less than 15 per cent of the population (Kenya, Uganda and Malawi in Africa, for example), fibre consumption is between 60 and 80 grams a day. Foods that contain fibre are filling, as we have stressed. This means that you are less likely to feel hungry in the two-hour period following a meal that contains large amounts of fibre.

Why is this the case? Fibre-containing foods add bulk and weight to the diet, and have been shown to have significant positive effects on weight loss when replacing fat. Fibre-containing foods release energy slowly into the bloodstream, giving the human body longer lasting, more sustained energy release than non-fibre-containing foods. This is beneficial in providing the body with what we consider to be good clean energy throughout the day. The role of fibre-containing foods, however, goes even further.

They interfere with the mixing of foods and digestive enzymes in the intestine in a positive way. Fibrous foods slow fat and carbohydrate absorption into the bloodstream. This is important for those seeking to lose weight because the slowing of fat absorption into the bloodstream means that you will feel fuller earlier and will therefore eat less food. The longer fat can stay in the intestine, the less likely you are to keep eating.

Of course we are not saying that you should eat a 250 gram block of chocolate followed by a bag of high-fibre prunes, but when fat intake is moderated, the addition of fibre can help prolong that feeling of satisfaction after a meal without a person having eaten large amounts of food. An excellent example is one-third of an avocado eaten as part of a healthy salad. The healthy fibre in the salad delays the fat of the avocado from entering the bloodstream, leaving you a little fuller than if you had eaten the avocado on its own.

High-fibre foods are low in fat (they virtually contain 0 grams of fat), low in energy and high in water content. Broccoli contains 4.1 grams of fibre for every 100 grams. This is considered to be a very significant amount of fibre. Eating an abundance of fibrous foods such as fruit, vegetables, brown rice, oats, legumes and nuts and seeds also gives us a feeling of health and wellbeing. This is undeniable. While many people refer to this as detoxing, it has more to do with just simply feeling in fantastic health.

If we were to look for a consistent pattern in helping us with weight loss, it would be to choose foods that contain large amounts of water as well as large amounts of fibre. No surprise then that fruit and vegetables fit this model perfectly.

Fat, carbohydrates and protein

Fat, carbohydrates and protein *all* contribute to the energy density of food. With carbohydrates and protein, we usually eat less of these before we begin to feel full. Imagine a piece of steak or a bowl of pasta. These are quite filling.

For the EDI to work successfully for your weight loss, you need to be aware that all of these macronutrients contribute to the energy of food you eat – even why they seem quite healthy and harmless.

Top 10 fibre-containing foods

1 wholemeal pasta
2 lentils
3 green peas
4 pear
5 sweet corn
6 rolled oats/muesli
7 banana
8 paw paw
9 broccoli
10 spinach

Where the EDI can help with weight loss

By now we are familiar with the term 'energy density', and understand what it is that makes a food energy dense. As we have pointed out there are many factors contributing to and increasing how much energy a food contains. Things like how much water a food has, how much fibre, fat as well as carbo-hydrates and protein are all important constituents of energy density. Understanding what energy density means will also help curb the volume of food we eat: eat less energy than your body expends in a given day.

The energy density of food is the most compelling tool in the fight against weight gain. It is at the forefront of obesity and weight management conferences, and if we are careful to consider the energy density of the food we eat, weight loss will happen quickly and easily. If you have been struggling with your weight, the EDI is the solution you have been looking for. If you have been buying low-fat products and believe you have been eating well most of the time and still cannot lose weight, you have undoubtedly not been considering the energy density of the food you are eating. Somehow the energy you have been consuming on a daily basis is outweighing the energy that your body uses. Let's see how you can correct this.

The EDI will help you:

- lose weight
- choose low energy dense foods
- make the best choice when comparing different fish, such as red and pink salmon, red meat, chicken or pork (ie. know which meat yields the least amount of energy per 100 grams)
- feel full after quite small amounts of food
- understand how much energy your body needs on a daily basis.

The EDI is a new way of ranking food according to the energy it contains. All foods are assigned a value from 0 to 100. The higher the EDI number, the more energy a food contains. A low EDI means food that is low in energy and good for you; a high EDI means food that is high in energy and bad for you. For example, a food that has an EDI of 5 has a very low amount of energy, but also more often than not has plenty of fibre and water, and is low in fat. A food that has a value of 60, which is considered a high number, means that this particular food is very high in energy and has plenty of fat and sugar and low amounts of water and fibre, and will ultimately lead to weight gain if consumed often enough.

The awesome fact about using the EDI is that all foods with low values are also low in fat, high in fibre, low in sugar and are enormously health giving. Following an eating plan consisting of 70–80 per cent low-to-moderate EDI foods guarantees substantial permanent weight loss. We have already seen this sustained by our clients over a two-year period. This permanent weight-loss is achieved chiefly by focusing on foods with an EDI of less than 20.

Broccoli, for example, with an EDI of 2 contains very little energy. The energy broccoli contains doesn't change a great deal regardless if it is boiled, steamed or raw. So, how you cook broccoli doesn't affect the EDI (although for some vegetables and fruit the EDI may change slightly with different cooking methods). Cheese has an EDI of 65, which is very high, and ties in with cheese's corresponding 1570 kJ of energy in a 100 gram slice. So beware – that 100 gram slice contains about 20 per cent of a woman's daily energy intake, and about 15 per cent of a man's. Imagine wasting 15 to 20 per cent of your energy intake for the day on a small piece of cheese!

It is no surprise that chocolate scores one of the highest EDI values of 100. We have made chocolate our reference food as it is the perfect high energy dense food, full of fat and sugar, with little water or fibre and massive amounts of energy per 100 grams. A 100 gram block (which is not actually such a big piece, when you think about it) contains 2200 kJ of energy and provides the average man and woman with 20 per cent and 28 per cent of their daily energy intake, respectively. The bad thing about getting our fuel from chocolate is that this energy is sluggish, relatively slow to be metabolised, and provides more energy than our body can use in a day.

FOOD (100 grams)	EDI	WATER (grams)	FAT (grams)	CARBOHYDRATE/ PROTEIN (grams)	FIBRE (grams)	ENERGY (kJ)
broccoli	2	88.7	0.3	5.3	4.1	137
cheese	65	41.4	32.4	20.4	0	1570
chocolate	100	1.5	32.4	61.6	0.5	2200

The Energy Density Index

All you need to remember is that the lower the EDI of a food, the lower the energy contained in the food. Consuming low to moderate EDI foods rather than high EDI foods will help you lose weight. We have divided food into five groups, according to their EDI as follows.

CATEGORY	EDI	RULES
1. Very low EDI foods	0–9	Eat plenty each day
2. Low EDI foods	10–19	Eat plenty each day
3. Moderate EDI foods	20–39	Eat 1–3 serves each day
4. High EDI foods	40–59	Eat occasionally
5. Very high EDI foods	>60	Eat once a week, or in small amounts

Each group contains many foods. This is the first complete comparison of foods with their corresponding energies. The EDI is a revolutionary tool that simplifies and enables weight loss. We have tabulated the most common foods here, but if there's something you can't find, please visit our web site for a more extensive list, or email us. For now let's investigate what foods are to be found in these groups. (All measurement are in grams and values are per 100 grams of food, unless marked, although the EDI of a food does not change if a larger quantity is eaten.)

Very low EDI foods: 0–9

The table following lists foods that are models of very low

EDI foods. Remember that the whole point of this book is to help you lose weight by consuming less energy than your body physically needs. This is a simple law of human metabolism and the core focus of losing weight.

The foods with EDI 0–9 contain low amounts of energy, between 0 and 400 kJ, and hence have a low EDI. The EDI is listed on the far left-hand side of the table. These foods, as characterised by broccoli (with an EDI of 2), are extremely low in fat, high in water and low in carbohydrates and protein. They are also high in fibre. All these foods have low amounts of energy.

Take a careful look now at some of the energy that various foods contain. Let's take a red apple and a green apple. A red apple contains only 205 kJ and has an EDI of 7, while the green apple has a little more energy at 224 kJ but has the same EDI of 7. This essentially means that the difference in energy is extremely small – not enough to affect the EDI.

Where possible we have listed the changes in both the EDI and energy of foods when they have undergone some kind of cooking. We have also tried to include different varieties of fruits and vegetables such as globe and Jerusalem artichokes, red and green capsicums, and red and green apples as well as brown and green pears. If a fruit or vegetable doesn't appear on our list or on our web site, please email us and we will add your food to our list.

Of course, eating or cooking any of these foods with oil, butter, cream, sugar or sour cream defeats the purpose of consuming a low energy dense food, as using any of these additives will add extra energy.

You may be surprised to see other foods included in the low EDI group, such as a beef casserole, low-fat milks and legumes such as lima beans. However, the beef casserole included here is full of vegetables and has a water base (see page 74), so per 100 grams it is a perfect low-energy dense food. Low-fat milk is also very water-based (93 grams of water per 100 grams) while lima beans, as with most legumes, absorb water when cooked. They are also low in fat and contain good amounts of fibre.

It is not necessary for you to analyse the energy content (kJ) of these foods as the most important thing here is to understand that their low EDI values indicate that these foods are low in energy and high in fibre.

In order to lose weight this group of foods should make up the bulk of your meals. (See pages 85–93 for the best meal suggestions using these foods.)

EDI	FOOD (100 grams)	WATER (grams)	FIBRE (grams)	FAT (grams)	CARBOHYDRATE/ PROTEIN (grams)	ENERGY (kJ)
1	lettuce	95.8	1.7	0.1	1.3	27
1	Chinese broccoli	91.8	3.7	0.1	3.5	93
2	spinach	93.5	2.7	0.3	3	85
2	cucumber	96.1	0.5	0.1	2.4	48
2	cabbage (boiled)	92.4	2.2	0	4.4	99
2	silverbeet (boiled)	93.2	3.3	0.1	3.7	65
2	fruit salad[a]	92.1	3.3	0.3	3.2	82

EDI	FOOD (100 grams)	WATER (grams)	FIBRE (grams)	FAT (grams)	CARBOHYDRATE/ PROTEIN (grams)	ENERGY (kJ)
2	strawberries	92.4	2.2	0.1	4.4	99
2	mixed vegetables[b]	90.7	2.8	0	5.1	106
2	zucchini	89	2.0	0.1	4.8	112
2	swede	92	2.8	0.1	5	110
2	broccoli (raw/ boiled/steamed)	88.7	4.1	0.3	5.3	137
2	asparagus (raw)	93.7	1.7	0.4	3.1	82
3	green capsicum (raw)	92.3	1.5	0.1	3.9	84
3	tomato	93.7	0.9	0.1	3.8	74
3	eggplant	94.7	1.2	0.1	3.9	56
3	green beans (boiled)	92.4	2.3	0.3	3.7	91
3	salad sandwich[c]	91.7	2.9	0.2	4.1	98
3	asparagus (cooked)	95.2	3	0.25	5.25	52
3	green capsicum (cooked)	91.4	1.5	0.1	4.4	91
3	globe artichoke	88.5	4.4	0.1	5.6	101
3	mushroom (raw)	92.3	1	0.1	5.2	99
3	watermelon	88.7	0.6	0.3	5.3	138
3	red capsicum (raw)	91.6	1.2	0.3	5.1	118
4	rockmelon	83	1	0.2	5.2	96
4	carrot	92.9	2.9	0.1	6.1	129
4	red capsicum (cooked)	83.4	2.5	0.2	7	228
4	mushroom (cooked)	91.1	1.2	0.2	5.9	117
4	orange (Valencia)	88.8	1.9	0.1	6.2	132
4	fig (fresh)	90	1.4	0.2	6.3	127
5	peach	88	1.4	0.1	7.3	143
5	mandarin	86.9	1.9	0.1	8.7	167
5	pineapple	85.9	2.5	0.3	8.1	169

EDI	FOOD (100 grams)	WATER (grams)	FIBRE (grams)	FAT (grams)	CARBOHYDRATE/ PROTEIN (grams)	ENERGY (kJ)
6	pumpkin	86	2.1	0.1	9	175
6	orange (navel)	88	2	0.1	9.1	172
6	cordial[d] (100 mL)	86.3	0	0.1	9.2	176
6	pea and ham soup[e]	92.6	0	0	9.7	157
6	pear (brown)	81	2.6	0.2	14.2	230
7	cherry	82.4	1.4	0.4	11.4	220
7	soy milk (low-fat)	88	0.9	1.3	7.4	182
7	apple (green)	82.5	1.7	0.2	10.4	224
7	parsnip	87.1	2.5	0.1	11.8	228
7	egg white	92.87	0	0.52	9.67	186
7	milk (low-fat)	93.24	0	0.4	10.85	175
7	rolled oats	85.1	1.9	0.1	11.1	199
7	cola	81	0	0	10.7	258
7	apple (red)	91.1	2	0.3	11.5	205
7	broad beans	68	5.6	0.7	13	371
8	freshly squeezed orange juice	87.3	0	0	12	204
8	pear (green)	76	4.2	0.5	13.4	278
8	eggplant (grilled)	85	1.2	0.1	12.3	204
8	mango	83	2.1	0.1	12.8	230
8	Jerusalem artichoke	84	2.3	0.1	12.9	229
9	sultana grapes	77.4	0.9	0.1	13.9	270
9	beef casserole[f]	71.1	7.2	0.5	17	308
9	lentils	73.7	3.7	0.4	15.8	321

(a) The fruit salad consists of rockmelon, watermelon, bananas, pineapple and mango.

(b) The vegetables include potato, pumpkin, carrot and zucchini, with no dressing or oil.

(c) A salad sandwich consists of tomato, carrot, cucumber

and lettuce, on wholemeal bread, no butter.

(d) The low EDI cordial can be any brand (full-strength, but we would recommend low-joule or sugar-free).

(e) The pea and ham soup is canned, any brand.

(f) The casserole is tomato-based and uses lean meat.

Low EDI foods: 10–19

The second table contains a list of foods and their EDIs that are still low and should form the basis of the foods consumed each day. The foods grouped in this bracket contain amounts of energy, ranging from 250 kJ to 550 kJ. The main difference in this group of foods compared to the foods we discussed in the 0–9 section is that they have a higher natural sugar or protein content, and a fractionally smaller fibre content.

Foods such as chickpeas and wholemeal pasta are included in this group due to their average, but not excessively high, amount of fibre and carbohydrate. When choosing foods to eat that won't impact on your weight, you cannot go past this group of foods, particularly when combined with the very low EDI foods on pages 54–56. They form a staple part of many diets around the world, where communities are generally lean and healthy. When consuming foods such as pasta or rice keep your serving sizes to one small to medium bowl (about the size of a woman's hand). (See also page 97 for ideal portion sizes.)

One question you may ask is whether it is possible to overeat foods in the first two groups (foods with an EDI of between 0–9 and 10–19)? One of the reasons that people are unable to eat massive amounts of these foods is that the fibre aids in providing the feeling of fullness. Casting our minds back to the section on fibre (see page 46), we said that our caveman ancestors ate between 77 and 120 grams of fibre daily. A quick calculation shows that this is an enormous amount of fruit and vegetables. This would be the same as eating six bananas, six apples and eight potatoes in one day. The more foods that you can consume from the first two groups (foods with an EDI of between 0 and 19), the more weight you will lose. So, even if you eat as much as you want, your energy intake will still be relatively low. Keep in mind, however, that you should avoid over-consuming pasta, rice, yoghurt or tuna, and always keep to the portion sizes that we have described in this book.

EDI	FOOD (100 grams)	WATER (grams)	FIBRE (grams)	FAT (grams)	CARBOHYDRATE/ PROTEIN (grams)	ENERGY (kJ)
10	potato (boiled)	80.2	1.9	0.1	14.8	256
10	regular milk	87	1.3	2.5	9.65	263
10	haricot beans	90.42	8.8	0.7	16.2	455
10	banana milkshake	80	1.1	0.2	15.6	272
11	jelly	73.8	0	0.4	17.3	294
11	red kidney beans	88.2	7.2	0.5	17	364
11	lima beans	82.8	5.3	0.3	17.7	335
11	yoghurt (low-fat)	82.2	0	0	17.3	283
12	yoghurt (no-fat)	78.9	0	0.2	17.9	315
13	chickpeas	60	5.7	0.1	21	565
13	rice (wild)	71.6	1.5	1	18.3	425
13	banana	75	2.2	0.7	20.8	377
13	yoghurt (full-cream)	78	0.1	4	20.5	369

EDI	FOOD (100 grams)	WATER (grams)	FIBRE (grams)	FAT (grams)	CARBOHYDRATE/ PROTEIN (grams)	ENERGY (kJ)
14	chicken and sweet corn soup	81.1	0	4.4	10.5	358
14	ham	72.8	0	2.7	24.2	511
16	baked beans	67	4.3	0.3	24.6	400
16	banana (sugar)	91	3.7	0.1	26.5	384
17	pasta (white)	70	1.8	0.3	26.8	500
17	soy beans	69	7.2	17	16	570
17	ham or tuna and salad sandwich	44.4	10	5	13.45	657
17	vegetarian lasagne	75.2	1.8	2.2	22.1	458
18	rice	69	0.8	0.2	28	523
18	pasta (wholemeal)	69	0.8	0.2	28	523
19	snapper (steamed)	74.1	0	5.1	16.8	487
19	tuna (canned in brine)	72	0	2.2	24.6	518

One of the great features of the EDI is that it allows us to compare foods and their properties that we were unable to before. This is clearly shown by comparing 100 grams of pasta, 100 grams of rice and 100 grams of tuna in brine; pasta and rice are carbohydrates, fish is protein. Whereas the Glycemic Index, for example, is not a useful tool for comparing fat, carbohydrates and protein as it is only a measure of a carbohydrate food, the EDI enables you to compare the characteristics of each of these macronutrients in relation to energy. While people continue to argue about carbohydrates versus proteins, the fact is they are very similar foods with respect to their energy characteristics. If we are primarily focusing on energy, then examine the profile of these foods carefully.

FOOD (100 grams)	ENERGY (kJ)	FAT (grams)	CARBOHYDRATE/ PROTEIN (grams)	FIBRE (grams)	EDI
pasta (cooked)	500	0.3	26.8	1.8	17
rice (cooked)	523	0.2	28	0.8	18
tuna (in brine)	518	2.2	24.6	0.0	19

The energy profiles of these foods are almost identical, as they all have very similar amounts of energy. The difference in energy between tuna (canned and packaged in brine) and rice is a mere 5 kJ. This is the same as a very thin slice of apple, so as you can see it isn't much. The amount of carbohydrates and protein they contain is almost the same, and this is fundamentally important as carbohydrates and protein contain the same amount of energy per gram of food. (The only difference, obviously, is that pasta and rice contain nearly all carbohydrate and fish all protein.) While the battle still rages between people fighting for either low-carbohydrate or high-carbohydrate diets, we now know that this is not the point at all, as both carbohydrates and protein contain the same amount of energy. The only way to promote weight loss is to focus on energy.

But let's look at why there is a difference between the pasta, which has an EDI of 17, and rice and tuna which have an EDI of 18 and 19 respectively. The first answer is fibre. Fibre is an integral part of the energy of a food, and the fibre in pasta is 1.8 grams in a 100 gram serving. As the abbreviated table above shows this is more than either rice or tuna which have 0.8 and 0 grams respectively. Looking back at the foods with EDI grouped from 0–9, you may remember that these foods have good amounts of fibre, which is one of the reasons that the energy density of these foods was low. Fibre helps to reduce the energy density of food. Secondly the tuna has more fat than either the rice or pasta. It has 2 grams more fat or (2 × 37.8) 76 kJ more energy from fat. This makes it a slightly more energy dense food than either pasta or rice, but not by much.

Moderate EDI foods: 20–39

The foods in this section have energies between 511 kJ and about 1000 kJ. Essentially these foods are protein based and you'll notice meat starting to appear. Using the EDI value of foods can extend your understanding of how various meats are different.

Foods from this group should be consumed regularly – at two meals a day (see specific meal suggestions on pages 85–93) – as protein is an essential nutrient for the body. These foods are higher in energy though, so the leaner the meat the lower the energy and hence the greater the weight loss that will be associated with this food selection. Foods with an EDI of less than 30 are still considered moderate in energy density. Foods with an EDI of greater than 30 in this group should be consumed less often than foods with an EDI less than 30. This forces people to make better food choices, opting for lean meats and cooking that involves removing skins and trimming excess fat.

Although cuts of lean beef are getting leaner, generally speaking, red meat has more fat than chicken, pork or veal. The exception here is chicken with the skin on. We all eat our chicken without skin now, don't we? (Fried chicken doesn't feature in this list as it has an EDI value of 51 – look for it in the high EDI group!)

This list of food also contains some values of fast foods. Some fast foods have similar energy to more common foods, but it is not intended for you to use the table to justify eating a sundae, just because a sundae has the same energy as a chicken and vegetable risotto. There are clear guidelines to make sure you always choose the healthier option. Keep in mind that the EDI is a way of choosing foods, but commonsense should also ensure you choose foods that are more nutritious, so after checking the EDI value, check the fat content and then the sugar in order to make a healthy choice.

The latter half of the table shows foods that are moving close to an EDI of 35 to 40. Apart from wholemeal bread products, these higher EDI foods, such as meat pies and sausages, should be eaten infrequently.

EDI	FOOD (100 grams)	WATER (grams)	FIBRE (grams)	FAT (grams)	CARBOHYDRATE/ PROTEIN (grams)	ENERGY (kJ)
20	low-fat ice-cream	60.7	0	0.8	30	546
21	meat lasagne	65.3	1.2	7.7	19	540
21	rice pudding	69.4	0.3	5.7	27	573
21	sorbet	64.9	0.2	0	33.5	539
21	spaghetti bolognaise	69	1.8	3.6	26.6	573
23	eggs	70.5	0.75	6.6	20.7	593
25	tuna pasta	65	1.2	6	20	539
25	sundae	67.9	0	6.1	23.7	630
26	chicken and vegetable risotto	75.1	0	11.2	12.6	627
27	baked potato (with oil)	60.5	0	5	29.4	660
27	chicken breast (roasted with no skin)	68.8	0	7	24.6	677
28	wholemeal crumpet (toasted)	47.3	4.4	0.1	45.9	834
31	lean beef (grilled)	63.5	0	6	35	838
32	full-cream ice-cream	41.2	0	11	23.3	1000
32	beef steak (grilled)	60	0	8.5	29	964
33	fillet steak (grilled)	60.9	0	9	29	849
34	mixed grain bread	38.7	4.8	2.9	54	1023
34	vanilla slice	58	0	10.6	26.3	850
34	wholemeal bread	39.2	6	1.2	54	993
34	minced steak	61.8	0	11.2	25.8	854
36	spaghetti marinara (cream-based)	50	1.8	15	20	927
37	white bread	44.4	2.9	2.6	53	990
37	meat pie	59.3	0	12.7	26	913
37	tuna (in oil)	61.5	0	13.7	24.4	922
38	fried sausage	63.7	0	16.1	19.3	924

We have included some of the data on fish, taken from several EDI tables, so you can get a closer look at how different fish compare to each other when it comes to their energy content.

Fish EDI

EDI	FOOD (100 grams)	WATER (grams)	FIBRE (grams)	FAT (grams)	CARBOHYDRATE/ PROTEIN (grams)	ENERGY (kJ)
15	cod	76.7	0	0.8	21	388
17	flounder	73.7	0	1.6	23.2	452
19	snapper	74.1	0	27	24	511
19	flathead	72.5	0	1.2	26.1	511
19	tuna (canned in brine)	72	0	2.2	24.6	518
22	trout	71	0	4.6	23.3	567
24	pink salmon	70.3	0	6.5	21.9	615
28	smoked salmon	68.1	0	4.6	32	561
33	red salmon	66.5	0	12	21.9	815
35	flounder (in batter, fried)	57	0.8	9.2	23	886
36	flathead (in batter, fried)	54.9	0.8	9	35	916

(All fish baked or steamed, unless otherwise stated.)

Note that the energy density and EDI change when fish is battered and fried, as opposed to steamed or baked. Flathead is a wonderful fish to eat, but when it's battered and then fried you add an extra 405 kJ of useless energy (to total 916 kJ) when you could have consumed only 511 kJ. How many people claim to have eaten 'only fish' for dinner, yet it was baked or fried in heaps of oil and the serving size was massive? If this is you, then think twice about the preparation of your food, or even the food that you are purchasing when you dine out and ask yourself if you are adding extra energy to your meals unnecessarily.

Snapper, for example, is a very lean fish and a good source of protein with little fat and a low amount of energy per 100 grams, hence it has an EDI of only 19. Eating foods such as snapper as part of your main meal will definitely aid in weight loss, especially if you prepare it baked or steamed.

But why do pink and red salmon have such different EDIs? The table shows they contain 615 kJ and 815 kJ of energy respectively. The difference in the energy of these pieces of fish is caused by the differing fat content of the two. Pink salmon has 6.5 grams of fat per 100 grams whereas red salmon has 12 grams, which results in a difference of 200 kJ. An analysis of meat, chicken and veal reveal that the redder the meat, the more fat and hence more energy a food contains.

High EDI foods: 40–55

Foods with EDI values between 40 and 55 contain plenty of energy. These foods should be eaten sparingly as they are not health-giving and do not promote weight loss, so we don't suggest trying to memorise all the EDI values here. It's just useful for you to see which foods fall into this group so you can avoid them.

In a single 100 gram serving of any of these foods the energy ranges from 932 kJ to 1960 kJ. As you are now well aware, this energy consumption is massive. To consume 100 grams of any food containing energy of this magnitude is surely not doing your weight any favours. Foods such as doughnuts, bacon, fried chicken and even corn flakes contain large amounts of fat and/or moderate amounts of carbohydrates and protein, which add up to a mass of energy. Comparing this list with the list of EDI foods between 0 and 9 shows a very dramatic energy difference. In the 0 to 9 EDI group, the energy content ranges from 100 to 300 kJ. Foods common to this group are those that we would normally eat on the run, or that we would consider to be fast food.

This is the area that we very often struggle with as these foods offer us comfort and convenience. The exception in this group of foods is raisins. Although the EDI of raisins is 45, no one really eats 100 grams of raisins. A handful at any time is going to be beneficial.

EDI	FOOD (100 grams)	WATER (grams)	FIBRE (grams)	FAT (grams)	CARBOHYDRATE/ PROTEIN (grams)	ENERGY (kJ)
41	jam	31	1.3	0	65.9	1080
41	marmalade	31.2	1.1	0	65.5	1056
45	French fries	42.9	1	16.1	31	1200
45	raisins	11.8	4.9	0.9	73	1259
50	bacon	40	0	27	36	1455
50	iced doughnut	57.1	0	23.2	45	1630
51	fried chicken (1½ pieces)	34.2	2.3	15.5	42	1780
52	honey	16.2	0	0	82.1	1320
53	corn flakes	3.3	0	0	82.1	1450
53	brown sugar	17	0	0	82.4	1448

Very high EDIs: More than 55

If you thought the foods in the last division of EDI values were high in energy, then foods with EDI values greater than 55 are surely at the pinnacle of energy density. These foods are laced with either massive amounts of fat or massive amounts of sugar or both. A single 100 gram serving of most of these foods packs an energy punch of between 1500–3700 kJ, potentially contributing 30 per cent of a person's daily energy requirements in that one serve.

As we have discussed, foods containing large amounts of fat are often smaller in size than foods that don't contain so much fat. This lethal combination of fat and sugar is what makes chocolate such an energy dense food. Chocolate is the standard by which all other foods are compared to in the synthesis of the Energy Density Index, and this is why chocolate has an EDI of 100. Foods such as butter, olive and sunflower oils have massive EDIs as they are pure fat and have whopping amounts of energy in them.

Eat these foods only very occasionally!

EDI	FOOD (100 grams)	WATER (grams)	FIBRE (grams)	FAT (grams)	CARBOHYDRATE/ PROTEIN (grams)	ENERGY (kJ)
60	chocolate éclair	44.5	0.8	1.2	91.6	1550
62	chocolate muffin	25.7	1.5	18.2	52.6	1563
65	cheese (common)	36.9	0	32.4	20.4	1570
66	coco pops	4.4	0.7	0.0	92	1563
70	Danish pastry with nuts and custard	23.4	1.8	24.5	49	1740
71	cream	51.9	0	42.8	4.8	1660

EDI	FOOD (100 grams)	WATER (grams)	FIBRE (grams)	FAT (grams)	CARBOHYDRATE/ PROTEIN (grams)	ENERGY (kJ)
77	salami (Hungarian)	34	0	37.6	23	1782
78	Snickers bar	5.4	6.7	25.6	62.1	2009
78	peanut butter	0.7	10.8	50	36	2520
86	chocolate biscuits	3.5	2.4	27.4	62.7	2069
87	potato chips	2.6	11.9	34	50	2195
88	popcorn	3.2	12.7	42.8	36	2348
88	white sugar	0.6	0	0	99.8	1597
89	corn chips	1.6	10	29	57	2160
99	peanuts	2.5	8	47.3	33.8	2388
100	CHOCOLATE	1.5	0.8	32.4	61.6	2200
118	cashew nuts	0.7	6.2	49.2	32	2400
118	sunflower oil	0.7	5.4	100	0	3040
130	butter	15.4	0	81.4	1	3050

Note that cashew nuts, butter, and oil have higher EDIs than our base value of 100 for chocolate. This is because in 100 grams there is a massive amount of energy in these foods. In practice, however, we'd hope that no one would be eating 100 grams of oil or butter in one sitting. Most of us would probably have a tablespoon of each, approximately 20 grams.

Cheese guide

As an addition to the table on high EDI foods, we thought it would be beneficial to analyse various types of cheese, so if people are going to splurge occasionally this table could at least help them to make a more informed decision. In the table on page 67 cheese has an EDI value of 65, which we chose as a good average value for common supermarket cheese, based on its nutritional information. However, a closer inspection shows that some soft cheeses, such as ricotta and cottage cheese, have medium EDI values, whereas the majority of the cheeses have values over 30.

EDI	FOOD (100 grams)	WATER (grams)	FIBRE (grams)	FAT (grams)	CARBOHYDRATE/ PROTEIN (grams)	ENERGY (kJ)
21	cottage cheese	75.4	0	5.8	17.6	512
25	ricotta	73.6	0	11.3	11.5	616
33	cheddar low-fat	50.3	0	7.2	34	844
34	goat's cheese	65	0	15.8	14.1	823
35	bocconcini	65.9	0	15.2	17.2	856
49	feta	52.2	0	23.3	18.1	1170
52	mozzarella	47.8	0	22	26.1	1260
54	camembert	51.6	0	26.3	18.7	1290
59	brie	48.6	0	29.1	19.4	1410
61	edam	38.8	0	27.2	28	1480
65	blue vein	41.4	0	32.4	20.4	1550
66	gouda	38.4	0	30.8	26.1	1590
66	Swiss	37.4	0	28.8	28.6	1600
70	cheddar	35.5	0	33.8	25.5	1690
70	Gloucester	36.5	0	34.3	25	1690
71	havarti	41.4	0	36.7	19.5	1690

Top 10 points to remember about energy density

1 Food portion sizes have increased both at home and in restaurants.

2 Larger food portion sizes lead to larger amounts

of energy being eaten, even when we are not hungry.

3 'Energy density' is the term used to describe how much energy food contains.

4 Foods high in water, such as fruit, have a low energy density.

5 Foods high in fibre usually have a low energy density.

6 Foods high in fat, such as cheese, have a high energy density

7 Foods that are high in both sugar and fat, such as chocolate and sweets, have a higher energy density.

8 The definition of a low energy dense food is one with low fat, low sugar, high water content and high fibre.

9 Low energy dense foods are more filling than high energy dense foods.

10 We eat much more food than we did a decade ago.

Summary

The best way to control the energy you consume is to follow the tables of EDI values in this chapter. In very simple terms, all foods have been ranked according to how much energy they contain. Foods with low values have low amounts of fat, carbohydrates and protein and are high in fibre. Foods that have high EDI numbers are foods that are either high in sugar or fat or both. Of all the work done in the field of obesity management and weight gain, the energy density of food remains the frontrunner in the fight against the bulge.

MAKING THE ENERGY DIET WORK FOR YOU

In this chapter you will learn:

- how to balance your energy intake for the day
- how not to overeat
- drinking a preload drink one to two hours before lunch and dinner can reduce the energy you consume during the day by 17 per cent
- soups, fruit and vegetables lower the energy density of food, due to the amount of water they contain

The EDI

Learning to use the EDI will assist you with weight loss. It is important that we all learn to use the EDI every time we eat, not just sometimes or when it's convenient. Ideally, you should follow it 24/7, but no one is perfect and trying to be is sometimes just too hard. If you take a day off once a week, don't despair; start again the next day with a clean slate. Use extra exercise to make up for small lapses (see also Chapter 7). Things are only difficult if we make them difficult, and successful when we decide to make them successful. Before continuing you need to decide if you have made your mind up to be successful.

This chapter focuses on how to use the EDI in order to facilitate weight loss. The theory behind the EDI is the result of investigating many healthy eating cultures, hundreds of medical journals and years of research. It requires that you take charge of the eating program, and use both this book and our web site as a source of valuable information (www.bpersonal.com.au). It is not necessary to memorise all the EDIs of foods (you can download them from our web site and stick them on your fridge), but rather be familiar with the characteristics of these foods. Keep in mind that the whole purpose of the EDI eating plan is for you to consume less of the wrong type of energy, and more foods with the correct form of energy, thereby eating less energy overall.

How to decrease the energy density of meals

When you are making a food choice always include foods that have these characteristics: low in fat and sugar, high in fibre, with a high water content. The water content of your food choices is extremely important (see page 44), and by including food that contains large amounts of water you allow your body to reach that feeling of fullness on a good weight of food, and good volume of food, largely stimulated by water. Hence including lots of foods such as soups, vegetables and fruits (which all contain over 90 per cent water by weight) in your diet, you are stimulating the volume receptors in your stomach, signalling to the brain the end of your hunger. Choose foods with EDIs of less than 20. Consuming 800 kJ less a day is important, as foods that contain large amounts of water have a lower kilojoule count than foods with little water. This means the energy density of your food is lower, leading you to not consume excess energy and so not gain weight.

Hint 1 *Add more water to your actual meals, not fat or oil*
Adding more water to your meals will actually reduce the amount of energy you consume. This is because you will feel fuller earlier and therefore won't eat as much.

Let's assume Jane's bowl of casserole, which contains beef and vegetables in a liquid base, contains 200 grams of food with an energy of 1000 kJ. This means that each 100 grams of food contains 500 kJ of energy (1000 kJ/2). So, we know that eating

200 grams of food will make Jane feel satisfied and trigger hunger to stop. If Jane adds 100 grams (ml) of water to her dish she now has 300 grams of food in her bowl. If she still eats 200 grams of food, the energy of the dish stays at 1000 kJ but she has diluted the energy per 100 grams. In other words by adding water to her dish, she now consumes more water and less energy (1000 kJ/3 = 333 kJ per 100 grams of food). Jane still eats a 200 gram portion of casserole, which contains 2 × 333 kJ = 666 kJ.

By adding water to your dish you now consume 333 kJ less energy per meal or 33 per cent less food, but still feel full. Of course, remember that the water needs to be added close to serving time to negate the effects of evaporation.

Adding fat or oil to your meal has the opposite effect to adding water. We touched upon this earlier saying that fat is less 'satiating' or filling, meaning it doesn't stimulate the brain to signal you have eaten sufficient. Let's see how it can increase the energy density of your meal. We call this 'passive over-consumption' of energy because people really don't understand that by adding such a little amount of oil, their energy intake can skyrocket.

Let's take the same 200 gram serving of casserole that contains 1000 kJ of energy. Instead of adding water Jane adds two tablespoons of oil. This is just a drop of olive oil in some people's eyes, but Jane has added 1300 kJ of energy to her meal. Remember, she was originally eating 1000 kJ in a 200 gram serve (500 kJ of energy per 100 grams serve). The total energy of her meal is now 1000 kJ + 1300 kJ = 2300 kJ – an immense increase. The weight of the meal has increased only slightly (200 grams + 36 grams of oil = 236 grams). If Jane still eats 200 grams of food, then for every 100 grams of food she eats she gets a whopping 974 kJ (2300/2.36) of energy. In her 200 grams of casserole she now eats 2 × 974 kJ = 1949 kJ of energy. She has increased the energy density of her meal by 949 kJ or an incredible 95 per cent. How on earth is she supposed to lose weight?

Comparing these changes in the energy density of both meals shows some startling differences. Jane has gone from a standard 1000 kJ meal and decreased it to 666 kJ, in the first case and increased it to 2300 kJ in the second case. The difference is 1634 kJ (or 389 calories). You should be able to see that anyone saving this much energy in one meal will surely lose weight. If you are adding extra energy to your meal instead of taking it away from your meal, how are you supposed to lose weight?

Of course, there's no need to be ridiculous about it or all your meals will be soup. This tool can come in handy to dilute soups, desserts such as jelly and in cooking in general.

Finally, what about actually drinking water with meals? For some unknown reason studies have not shown the same changes to energy density as when water is incorporated into food. By all means drink water with your meals (or even better, try a preload, see page 94), but don't substitute a glass of water for cooking with extra water.

Hint 2 *Add beans such as cannellini, red kidney, soy and lima beans to your meals*

Adding beans lowers the EDI and increases the nutritional value of your meal. Flavour can be further improved through the addition of herbs and spices, or tomatoes instead of water (as the water they contain is sufficient).

Peter makes a meal of pasta with canned tomatoes, pasta sauce, onions and mince meat. He is cooking for five people. Again let's assume that each serve of pasta contains 200 grams of food and has 1000 kJ of energy. So, in Peter's saucepan there is enough food for five people (5 × 200 grams = 1000 grams or 1 kg, and 5 × 1000 kJ = 5000 kJ). If Peter adds 400 grams of cannellini beans, which contain only 1520 kJ, his cooking pot now contains 1400 grams of food (the original 1000 grams plus 400 grams of beans). The energy of the food in his pot is now 6520 kJ (the original 5000 kJ and 1520 kJ from the beans).

Before adding the beans each 100 grams of food equals 500 kJ of food, hence 200 grams has 1000 kJ. By adding beans, which contain 70 per cent of their weight as water and fibre, and have an EDI of only 12, Peter lowers the energy density of each 100 grams of food to 465 kJ, and hence the total 200 gram serving that each person gets is now 931 kJ. This is a saving of about 70 kJ per meal.

What works even better for Peter is when he adds an extra 300 grams of water to his dish. His pot now contains the same 6520 kJ of energy and the weight would be 1700 grams. Per

100 grams of food Peter has now further reduced the energy density to 383 kJ and for the 200 gram serve each person gets 766 kJ, a total saving of 234 kJ. This is significant. If Peter saves 234 kJ for three meals during the day, he saves 704 kJ per day, and nearly 5000 kJ per week.

If Peter adds oil to his dish instead (in the order of four to five tablespoons) to give his dish more taste, he adds only 90 grams of weight, but 3750 kJ of energy. He increases the energy density of his meal per 200 gram serving to a massive 1600 kJ. This increases the energy density of each meal by 60 per cent.

Hint 3 *Add vegetables to your meals*

Karen is cooking risotto with chicken for her family of five. Each 200 gram serving contains 1000 kJ of energy. This means that in her cooking pot there is 5×200 g = 1000 grams of food and 5×1000 kJ = 5000 kJ of energy. By adding vegetables to the dish, Karen can dramatically alter the energy density of her family's meals.

Karen adds 500 grams of vegetables to the pot and only 725 kJ of energy. Her pot now contains 1500 grams of food and 5725 kJ of energy. She chooses the vegetables shown in the following table. Note that all the vegetables are characterised by their low EDI. These low EDI values indicate that these foods have low amounts of energy, high fibre and can help if incorporated into a meal to reduce the energy density of a meal. Per 100 grams these foods contribute about 80 to 90 per cent water by weight and very little energy. They also contribute greatly to the vitamin and mineral needs of the body.

VEGETABLES (100 grams)	EDI	WATER (grams)	ENERGY (kJ)
broccoli	2	89	137
zucchini	2	89	112
green beans	3	92	91
carrots	4	93	129
potato	10	80	256

Karen adds weight to her meal without adding energy. This is one of the best features of the EDI – and the main reason it works for permanent weight loss. For each 100 grams in her pot there is now only 382 kJ, reduced from 500 kJ (1500/15 = 100 grams, therefore 5725 kJ/15 = 382 kJ per 100 grams). This means that each person gets 763 kJ per 200 gram serve or bowl – a saving of 236 kJ for the meal.

Hint 4   *Add salad to sandwiches*

Jim purchases a takeaway ham and cheese roll for lunch, which weighs about 170 grams and contains 1600 kJ of energy. In every 100 grams of ham and cheese roll there is 1600/ 1.7 = 942 kJ of energy. This is a large amount of energy – not surprising considering cheese has an EDI of 65. If Jim asks for some salad in his roll instead of cheese, he adds 350 grams of weight and only 307 kJ of energy to his bread roll and ham. His new ham and salad roll weighs 470 grams with a corresponding energy of 1150 kJ. This is much less energy than his original ham and cheese roll (1600 kJ). And his bread roll looks bigger as it is stuffed with so much salad, compared to his flat ham and cheese roll. Per 100 grams of food his ham and salad roll has only 269 kJ. Adding vegetables to any sandwich or roll can also reduce the energy density of your food and, like Jim, you could save yourself 450 kJ a day by doing something that seems almost too simple.

SALAD	EDI	WATER (grams)	ENERGY (kJ)
cucumber (50 g)	2	48	24
spinach leaves (50 g)	2	42	43
tomato slices (150 g)	3	141	111
grated carrot (100 g)	4	93	129

Hint 5 *Drink soups as many times as possible during the week – once a day if you can*

Soups are already very full of water so most of the time people are going to feel full much earlier than normal because the volume of food they consume is large. This means less energy!

In hot climates where eating soup is not always possible or practical, try to have a salad instead, at least once a day.

Hint 6 *Try rice noodle soups*

The Vietnamese have the right idea as they eat a lot of rice noodle soups. These are essentially a clear broth with either chicken or red meat, plenty of fresh vegetables and rice noodles. This is such a filling dish with the noodles, vegetables and fluid. If you cannot get to a Vietnamese restaurant, learn how to make rice noodle soup from scratch, it really is quite easy.

Hint 7 *Add only salt for flavour instead of high energy-dense additives*

Rather than add oil, butter, margarine, cream, ghee or lard to your cooking, simply add a little salt for taste. As you have seen in our previous examples, just a little oil can add a hefty amount of energy to your meal. Use low-fat milk as a substitute for cream in sauces and soups, or use water instead, if possible.

Hint 8 *If you've eaten less energy from a main meal, don't undo all your good work*

You've seen how our friends have tried and succeeded to reduce the energy content of their meals. There is no point reducing the energy intake of your meals if you're then going to sit in front of the TV for the rest of the evening and gobble down a block of chocolate. This may sound extreme, but it's actually very common. We know that lots of people do this because they tell us so in their emails! There is little logic in saving 700 kJ from dinner if you then consume another 2000 kJ or more with chocolate or biscuits or sweets just as an after-dinner treat. Now you know it is silly to blame the potatoes for your weight problem, or the bread, when you haven't been honest with yourself about your hidden stash of chocolate.

Hint 9 *Try to cook at home most nights*

If you cook at home you know exactly how much energy is in your meal. In a restaurant or café it is much harder to tell how something has been cooked. Even when a salad or muffin looks quite healthy, there can be all kinds of hidden energy boosters – dressings, oils, sugars. Don't ruin your social life just so you can lose weight, but be aware of what you might be eating when you're not making the meal yourself. (See also Chapter 5 on restaurant and takeaway food.)

Hint 10 *Eat lots of fruit – at least 5 pieces a day*
Fruit fills you up while being very low on the EDI scale. It's full of fibre and essential nutrients and vitamins.

Handy hints

When cooking, incorporate the following steps to maximise your weight loss using the EDI approach.

1   Add water to your meals (e.g. casseroles, pasta, risotto or other foods).

2   Add vegetables and legumes to your cooking. These too will contribute water and weight to your meals without the extra energy.

3   Avoid using oil or cheese where possible. They contribute little water, plenty of weight and hundreds of times the energy that fruit, vegetables and water do.

4   Always make foods with low EDIs the dominant foods on your plate.

By following these basic rules you will decrease your energy intake by as much as 15 to 40 per cent per meal. Some people may only need to decrease the amount of daily energy intake by about 15 per cent, which doesn't seem like much, but if you are eating only 15 per cent more energy than your body burns, then reducing energy by this amount is sufficient. A decrease of such a small amount of food should not be underestimated and can be very significant when it comes to shedding weight.

Energy eating plans
The response and feedback from numerous people who have been trialling these meal suggestions for breakfast, lunch and

dinner have been very positive. The most common response was a feeling of being energetic yet feeling light, which is exactly what we wanted to achieve. This is such a change from how we normally feel – flat and lethargic.

If you feel full at the end of any meal, you need to cut back on your portion size. The chances are that if you feel full you have consumed more energy than your body needs. This will be your greatest challenge, as the body's natural instinct is to gorge. Portion sizes are often the trickiest thing to get right. The responses to our own studies suggest that small to medium portion sizes should fill most people up. But we recommend that you use smaller plates and bowls to resist the temptation of overeating. It's amazing how some of our male clients claimed to be eating a small meal when in fact the bowl was the size of a dinner plate, and the food in the actual bowl was enough to feed a family of four.

The main idea behind the EDI is to encourage all people to eat the majority of foods with EDI values of less than 20. Eat 70–80 per cent of your foods from the list of under 20 EDI, 15 per cent of foods from 20 to 40 EDI and 5 per cent of foods over 40 EDI. Remember to keep the portions small, especially for those foods with a value over 40. This way, you can eat a small piece of chocolate without feeling too guilty. If you can follow this simple guideline, where with every meal you have very low EDI value foods, then you should finally begin to see the weight fall away.

The Top 10 low energy dense meals

The following breakfasts, lunches and dinners have been designed to provide you with enough energy for your day, from the right types of foods, without overloading your body with too much energy.

As you become familiar with the pattern of eating, we encourage you to create your own low energy dense breakfasts, using the EDI as a guide. Notice that all the foods have essentially low to medium EDI values. Although some values in the meal plan are higher, such as that of wholemeal bread (34), in reality you are only eating two pieces of bread, which in no way provide too much energy. If you cannot find the EDI for a food, please visit our website.

BREAKFAST 1	EDI	ENERGY (approx.)
rolled oats (150 grams)	7	318 kJ
low-fat milk (100 ml)	7	175 kJ
5 strawberries	2	59 kJ
Total energy = 552 kJ (131 calories)		

BREAKFAST 2	EDI	ENERGY
low-fat, low-sugar muesli (100 grams)	34	450 kJ
low-fat milk (100 ml)	7	175 kJ
Total energy = 625 kJ (150 calories)		

BREAKFAST 3	EDI	ENERGY
banana milkshake (with 300 ml milk, yoghurt and banana)	10	900 kJ
Total energy = 900 kJ (214 calories)		

BREAKFAST 4	EDI	ENERGY
tropical fruit salad (400 grams)	2	328 kJ
natural low-fat yoghurt (100 grams)	11	233 kJ
Total energy = 611 kJ (145 calories)		

BREAKFAST 5	EDI	ENERGY
ham (100 grams) (pan-fried, no oil)	14	511 kJ
1 tomato (pan-fried, no oil)	3	84 kJ
wholemeal toast (1 slice)	34	413 kJ
Total energy = 1088 kJ (240 calories)		

BREAKFAST 6	EDI	ENERGY
ham (100 grams)	14	511 kJ
1 tomato	3	84 kJ
1 egg (ham, tomato and egg pan-fried with no oil)	23	316 kJ
wholemeal toast (1 slice)	34	413 kJ
Total energy = 1324 kJ (315 calories)		

BREAKFAST 7	EDI	ENERGY
rice pudding (200 grams)	21	1146 kJ
5 strawberries	2	59 kJ
Total energy = 1205 kJ (286 calories)		

BREAKFAST 8	EDI	ENERGY
wholemeal toast (1 slice)	34	413 kJ
strawberry jam (1 tablespoon)	41	150 kJ
low-fat milk or soy (400 ml)	7	728 kJ
Total energy = 1291 kJ (307 calories)		

BREAKFAST 9	EDI	ENERGY
wholemeal toast (1 slice)	34	413 kJ
1 egg	23	316 kJ
low-fat milk or soy (300 ml)	7	577 kJ
Total energy = 1306 kJ (311 calories)		

BREAKFAST 10	EDI	ENERGY
wholemeal crumpets (1–2)	28	515 kJ
marmalade (1 tablespoon)	41	150 kJ
low-fat milk or soy (400 ml)	7	728 kJ
Total energy = 1393 kJ (332 calories)		

LUNCH PRELOAD	EDI	ENERGY
low-fat high-calcium milk or soy (500 ml)	7	985 kJ
2 pieces of fruit	5	550 kJ
Total energy = 1535 kJ (365 calories)		

LUNCH 1	EDI	ENERGY
wholemeal toast (2 slices)	34	820 kJ
1 tomato, chopped, with basil	3	86 kJ
½ rockmelon	4	280 kJ
Total energy = 1186 kJ (282 calories)		

LUNCH 2	EDI	ENERGY
pea and ham soup (canned, 200 grams)	6	464 kJ
½ honeydew melon	4	408 kJ
Total energy = 872 kJ (207 calories)		

LUNCH 3	EDI	ENERGY
roast beef (3 slices)	31	225 kJ
1 large potato	10	400 kJ
1 banana	13	537 kJ
Total energy = 1162 kJ (277 calories)		

LUNCH 4	EDI	ENERGY
minestrone soup (200 ml)	7	500 kJ
wholemeal bread (1 slice)	34	413 kJ
2 oranges	6	468 kJ
Total energy = 1381 kJ (329 calories)		

LUNCH 5	EDI	ENERGY
roast beef (3 slices)	25	225 kJ
wholemeal bread (2 slices)	34	820 kJ
watermelon (400 grams)	3	550 kJ
Total energy = 1595 kJ (380 calories)		

LUNCH 6	EDI	ENERGY
steamed chicken breast (100 grams)	27	853 kJ
salad (200 grams)	3	130 kJ
bunch of grapes (100–150 grams)	9	300 kJ
Total energy = 1283 kJ (305 calories)		

LUNCH 7	EDI	ENERGY
salad sandwich	3	1026 kJ
1 pear	6	200 kJ
1 mandarin	5	185 kJ
Total energy = 1411 kJ (336 calories)		

LUNCH 8	EDI	ENERGY
vegetable soup (200–300 ml)	7	500 kJ
wholemeal bread (1 slice)	34	413 kJ
2 apples	7	782 kJ
Total energy = 1695 kJ (403 calories)		

LUNCH 9	EDI	ENERGY
tuna (canned in brine, 180 grams)	19	824 kJ
wholemeal bread (2 slices)	34	820 kJ
2 oranges	6	501 kJ
Total energy = 2145 kJ (511 calories)		

LUNCH 10	EDI	ENERGY
½–1 salmon sandwich	30	1034 kJ
large salad (400 grams)	3	300 kJ
watermelon (400 grams)	3	550 kJ
Total energy = 1884 kJ (436 calories)		

DINNER PRELOAD	EDI	ENERGY
600 ml–1 L water or	0	0
600–700 ml low-fat milk/soy milk	8	1100 kJ
banana (small)	13	380 kJ
apple	7	380 kJ
Total energy = 2116 kJ (503 calories)		

DINNER 1	EDI	ENERGY
vegetable soup (200–300 ml)	7	500 kJ
wholemeal bread (1 slice)	34	413 kJ
watermelon (400 grams)	3	550 kJ
Total energy =1463 kJ (348 calories)		

DINNER 2	EDI	ENERGY
vegetable lasagne	17	1129 kJ
(1 medium slice, 200 grams)		
jelly (small bowl, 100 grams)	11	294
Total energy = 1423 kJ (339 calories)		

DINNER 3	EDI	ENERGY
tuna pasta (no oil) (200 grams)	25	1120 kJ
salad (400 grams)	3	300 kJ
Total energy = 1420 kJ (340 calories)		

DINNER 4	EDI	ENERGY
beef and vegetable casserole (200 grams)	9	1250 kJ
low-fat ice-cream (2 small scoops)	20	237 kJ
Total energy = 1487 kJ (354 calories)		

DINNER 5	EDI	ENERGY
baked fish (150 grams)	17	665 kJ
baked assorted vegetables (300 grams)	2	325 kJ
fruit salad (500 grams)	2	500 kJ
Total energy =1659 kJ (378 calories)		

DINNER 6	EDI	ENERGY
baked beans (100–150 grams)	16	1060 kJ
wholemeal toast (2 slices)	34	820 kJ
salad (200 grams)	3	160 kJ
Total energy = 2040 kJ (485 calories)		

DINNER 7	EDI	ENERGY
chicken and vegetable risotto (200 grams)	26	1230 kJ
fruit salad (500 grams)	2	500 kJ
Total energy = 1730 kJ (411 calories)		

DINNER 8	EDI	ENERGY
spaghetti bolognaise (200 grams)	21	1000 kJ
steamed vegetables (400 grams)	2	450 kJ
sorbet (2 medium scoops)	21	430 kJ
Total energy = 1880 kJ (447 calories)		

DINNER 9	EDI	ENERGY
chicken breast (pan-fried, no oil)	27	1175 kJ
vegetables (lightly pan-fried, no oil)	2	450 kJ
rice (50 grams)	18	250 kJ
low-fat ice-cream (2 small scoops)	20	237 kJ
Total energy = 2112 kJ (401 calories)		

DINNER 10	EDI	ENERGY
baked chicken breast (medium)	27	1175 kJ
baked/steamed vegetables (400 grams)	2	450 kJ
mango (100 grams)	8	236 kJ
Total energy = 1861 kJ (443 calories)		

The importance of preloads

Preloads as their name suggests are pre-meal drinks/food that are consumed in the one to three hours prior to a meal, usually between meals. Preloads work extremely well from a scientific viewpoint, resulting in people eating 17 per cent less food during a typical day. Our own data shows that with our eating plans, preloads mean a 30 per cent reduction in energy consumed for a day.

For women and men, respectively, this means approximately 1360 kJ (323 calories) and 2000 kJ (465 calories) less energy per day. Once again the preloads can be water-based and work on the principle of a person consuming a certain volume of food each day, which in turn stimulates the receptors in the stomach to signal the brain to cease eating. The added weight of water-containing foods helps with this process.

With these preloads you may actually find that you eat less food during lunch and dinner. Men may prefer to consume 600 to 700 mL of low-fat milk/soy for dinner preloads rather than water if they find they are getting hungry. Dinner preloads should also contain some fruit, but if you have opted to drink milk then don't eat citrus fruits as this could result in an upset stomach.

Calcium and iron

Two minerals that are essential to the human body functioning well are calcium and iron. Without these two vital minerals we all, but especially women, run the risk of anemia and osteoporosis. Each day we need 800 mg of calcium and 12 to 16 mg of iron. Calcium can be obtained from: three glasses of milk (750 mg calcium), 200 g of low-fat yoghurt (350 mg calcium), salmon and sardines, 100 grams (containing 250 mg and 330 mg respectively), 50 g of cottage cheese (200 mg). Iron can be found in green leafy vegetables, such as spinach and lean meat (two slices contain 2 to 2.5 mg). Keep this in mind when choosing your foods.

Food choices

In total women should aim for an energy intake of approximately 6000 kJ and men about 9000 kJ per day. Of course we are not saying that you need to eat exactly 6000 kJ or 9000 kJ but you should aim for this. If you eat around 200–400 kJ over, it is not going to ruin your day. If your energy intake exceeds this even further then you have tipped your energy balance, resulting in your body storing extra energy.

Putting all the science from this book into action shows that if you eat approximately 6000 kJ for the day and then eat either 5 grams of fat or 5 grams of carbohydrate you would be eating an extra 189 kJ or 84 kJ, respectively. Although both fats and carbohydrates have the same weight, fat has more than double the energy of carbohydrates so you are more likely to overconsume when eating fat than when eating carbohydrates. If your job means you sit down all day, then you certainly don't need extra energy. You need enough to get you through the day and some left over at night. Eating more energy than your body needs will lead to weight gain.

One of the challenges people face is that when a menu plan states one salmon roll, people will often eat two or one oversized one. The other problem is they follow the plan, but add their own snacks such as a sweet biscuit or a chocolate bar, which throws everything out the window, especially when you are trying to control your energy intake. If you know you're going to snack on something that's not on the plan, then choose the meals with the lowest amounts of energy during the day, such as Breakfast 1, Lunch 8 and Dinner 4. This will yield only 4000 kJ for the day, and with your lunch and dinner preloads and even a small piece of chocolate you should end up with 6000 kJ, which is still a good day's work. However, if you do well with all your meals and then throw in a 200 gram chocolate bar, you are adding 4300 kJ extra to your day. This is a massive energy intake and will never lead to even the remotest amount of weight loss. Let's not kid ourselves that we are only eating chocolate for the antioxidants. For the chocolate addicts who still want to decrease their weight we hope this provides you with some alternative and some hope.

How do I know exactly how much energy I am eating each day?

It is very difficult to calculate exactly how much energy you eat each day. You could do this by weighing foods and using a calorie counter, but who has time to do this? By understanding the relationship that food has with energy and how large portion sizes also contribute to our energy intake and hence weight, you will be able to reduce the unnecessary energy you eat. By adding water to your meals (such as soups and casseroles), as well as drinking water-based drinks (such as milk and water itself), you will consume the right amount of energy without having to think about counting calories.

Portion sizes

One of the biggest factors here is the size of the plates and bowls we use. Use smaller plates and bowls than you're used to! Here is a list of some good food portion sizes that you may find handy. These are what we recommend.

FOOD	SERVING SIZE
fruit salad	a handful
piece of fruit	a tennis ball
vegetables	a large handful
rice, pasta, potatoes	1–1½ handfuls
1 slice of bread	
foccacia	2 open hands
soup	a large bowl, particularly if water-based
red meat	a tennis ball
chicken	an audio cassette
fish	a hand
pancake	a CD
muffin	a tennis ball
cake	a tennis ball
chocolate	an index finger
soft drink	a styrofoam cupful
cup of coffee/tea	a tennis ball
beer	a styrofoam cupful

Being more accountable

When we sit down to eat we must understand that when we go back for second and third serves of food the chances are it's not because we are hungry. The fact that food is within arm's reach leads us to eat. Do we need this energy? The chances are we don't, especially during days of inactivity. Following a diet plan is one thing, but doubling the serves on the menu plan will put your energy intake way over your daily limit.

Millions of people worldwide are questioning what they are eating, but as the medical studies show it is not so much *what* that matters as *how much*. Recall that the size of the steak on your plate is 225 per cent greater in size than it should be. A piece of meat should be about the size of your palm, not the size of the plate. Serves of pasta are 400 per cent greater than recommended. The pasta isn't bad for you, but is having three bowls going to aid in the reduction of weight? Surely not.

When purchasing food from the supermarket, take the time to read the labels and choose lower energy foods. As consumers we need to understand as best as we can what we are putting in our mouths. You wouldn't want to give harmful foods to your pets, so why would you neglect checking what is going in your mouth?

Summary

The meals that have the lowest energy (those with a low EDI), are based around soup, fruit and vegetables, since these foods are very high in water. Remember the water in food dilutes the energy in your meal just as water dilutes sweet cordial. This means lowered amounts of energy are consumed, although the same weight of food may be eaten, leading to an energy deficit.

With some very simple steps you will be able to reduce the energy density of your meals drastically – and then you will see significant changes in your weight. It is that easy.

WHAT YOU CAN DO ABOUT ALCOHOL AND EATING OUT

In this chapter you will learn:

- alcohol consumption prevents the body from burning fat, reducing fat burning by 80 per cent
- alcohol is slow to be metabolised
- alcohol is usually consumed with high energy dense fat, pushing the human body further into fat storage
- restaurant foods are very energy dense with most serves having high EDI values
- eating low EDI foods as an entree can lead to reductions in energy intake and hence weight loss

Your social life

What happens when we go out? How do we control our energy intake if we have a business lunch in a restaurant or attend a friend's party at the local pub?

We've been told that it's okay to eat most foods as long as we eat them in moderation. But when was the last time you ate in moderation when you were at a restaurant? Probably never? Why? Moderation doesn't come into our thoughts when we dine out or grab some takeaway, because what dominates our thoughts is 'value for money', a common theme of this book and a common theme in the etiology of energy density and weight gain. There is also the social and even cultural aspect of dining out. When the party is in full swing and after a glass or two of red, you say to yourself, the diet starts on Monday. You're out to have fun, and cutting back or cutting down on food is not fun!

So, once again consider the last time you ate in moderation when you dined out at a restaurant. Did it mean that you ate so much that you could barely walk, or did it mean that you just didn't go back for your third helping of food? Did it mean that you ate less food but made up for it in the alcohol department, drinking four glasses of red wine instead of two? Did it mean that you ate less but instead drank three stubbies of beer instead of two?

Drink and be merry – alcohol metabolism

One of the great joys of life is to have a drink with friends, celebrate an occasion, or have a relaxed drink with dinner.

Although there are numerous reputable studies that suggest that having a drink is actually beneficial to our hearts, we need to watch we don't overdo it. Too much of a good thing can become harmful to our health and causes weight gain. Every time a study about the health benefits of a glass of alcohol appears it tends to reinforce people's excuse to drink: if one glass is good, three must be even better.

But have you ever wondered how having just one drink, which we know is good for our health, impacts on fat metabolism? Have you ever stopped to consider that even two standard drinks of alcohol may impact in a negative way when it comes to weight loss? Would it surprise you to know that we have had great weight-loss results, 40 kilograms or more, just from people cutting out their alcohol consumption?

First, let's remember that 1 gram of alcohol has more energy than either 1 gram of carbohydrate or 1 gram of protein (see page 48). For each gram of alcohol there is 29.4 kJ of energy. Alcohol doesn't require any digestion so it is quickly absorbed from our stomachs and small intestine. Most people will tell you that alcohol then gets converted to fat. This is incorrect, and as analysis techniques have become very advanced in only the last few years it has allowed us the luxury to 'see' what happens to alcohol. Only 5 per cent gets converted to fat. Relief, you may say! If you consume only two drinks, which contain 24 grams of alcohol, then only 1.2 grams of this gets converted into fat. What happens to the other 95 per cent of the alcohol in our two drinks?

Alcohol is converted to a substance called acetate in the liver and then released into the bloodstream. In fact 80 per cent of the alcohol you drink is converted to acetate. From our two drinks, nearly 19 grams would be re-released into the blood stream as acetate, over a period of a few hours, as alcohol can only be broken down at about 10 grams per hour. This acetate then travels to the muscles where it is burned as fuel for moving muscles.

This all sounds quite simple, but the real problem is that acetate is a potent inhibitor of the release of fat from our fat cells. When acetate enters the blood stream, lipolysis (the release of fat from fat cells) is ceased. To make matters even more unfavorable, when acetate is released into the blood stream, any fat already in the blood (which is being used for muscles and tissues around the body for energy) is pushed back into fat cells. The result is that when we drink alcohol we burn a lot less fat. Up to 60 per cent less fat enters the blood stream, and the body decreases using body fat by 80 per cent, and instead of burning body fat for energy, the body burns the alcohol byproduct acetate.

Some studies show that the decrease in the use of fat for energy is almost balanced by the body's burning of acetate. In understanding this, we understand that the type of energy we want our body to burn for weight loss is important. We certainly don't want energy from alcohol being burnt at the expense of energy from fat, carbohydrate or protein!

Having the body burn acetate (energy from alcohol) instead

of burning energy from fat from our body's fat stores means we are clearly consuming the wrong type of food, resulting in the body burning the wrong type of energy. Burning energy from alcohol instead of from fat will only lead to an enhanced weight gain. This process continues until all the alcohol is used, and it can take over 10 hours for a big night, depending on how much you drink. Despite this new use of acetate for energy, the body still burns carbohydrate. In fact the amount of carbohydrate found in the blood (as glucose) doesn't change while alcohol is being metabolised.

This means there are a number of practical considerations for the person trying to lose fat and weight. The human body can metabolise only a certain amount of alcohol per hour. In approximate terms this boils down to 7 to 14 grams per hour for an 80 kilogram man and 6 to 12 grams per hour for a 60 kilogram woman. This sounds fine in theory, but in reality it's quite slow.

TYPE OF DRINK (standard sizes)	AMOUNT (ml)	ALCOHOL CONTENT (ethanol) (grams)	STANDARD DRINKS
beer (low alchohol) 1 can	375	8	0.8
beer 1 glass	210	8	0.8
beer 1 can	375	14	1.4
beer 1 bottle	750	28	3
wine 1 glass (small)	60	8	0.8
spirits	30	9	0.9

The social setting of alcohol consumption is usually at a bar or a restaurant, and this further decreases the body's ability to burn fat, as you will see. You're eating restaurant food or potato chips, nuts and fast food, and the body is pushed further into energy storage, and not into energy use. As you will see in our analysis of restaurant food, it is very common to eat large amounts of fat, hence large amounts of energy, as well as medium amounts of alcohol, and then leave a restaurant with the human body four to six hours behind in its fat metabolism process.

Restaurant food is a huge 'unknown' in terms of energy, and weight gain, and it is almost always coupled with alcohol consumption. Even when you try to select the most healthy seeming options on the menu, your really have no idea of how much energy you are eating and drinking. We have found amazing weight-loss success with people who simply eat more often at home, and cut restaurant and takeaway food from two to three times a week to once a week. With this decreased consumption of restaurant food, we also find a marked decrease in alcohol consumed for the week. Many people claim that they eat well and don't know why they put on weight. Many forget to account for alcohol consumption. Do you claim you cannot lose weight yet find yourself with a menu in your hands two to three times a week? The chart on page 106 shows how alcohol and restaurant food can each add another third to your daily energy intake. *Note:* The food figures in this chapter are actual examples and may differ from standard servings.

ALCOHOL AND ENERGY INTAKES

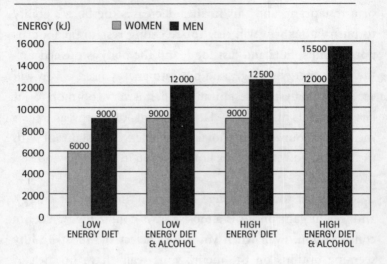

ENERGY (kJ) ☐ WOMEN ■ MEN

A person trying to lose weight can eat well during a typical week and consume a low amount of energy, which is conducive to weight loss, by eating foods with a low to moderate EDI. But while following this pattern of eating, many people still consume alcohol. Even two to three drinks two to three times a week have a huge impact on energy and slow the use of body fat, as you can see in the table above.

As this clearly shows a woman can increase her energy from a weight-losing 6000 kJ to a weight-gain, fat-storing 9000 kJ just by adding a couple of drinks of alcohol. A man too can undo all his good work from a weight-losing 9000 kJ to a weight-gaining 12 000 kJ. This type of eating is almost identical to the high energy, high fat eating, which you can see yields almost the same amounts of energy. This shows that there is little point eating well and then drinking, as the energy you consume through the alcohol makes up for the energy you don't eat during the week. While people are blaming bread, rice, fat and all sorts of other things for weight gain, few have recognized that alcohol is a huge player.

Of course, you can see that a high energy diet coupled with large alcohol consumption can lead to 12000 kJ of food per day for women and 15500 kJ of food eaten for men. This is horrendously high and will keep the body from burning fat for many hours, storing fat instead.

The biggest challenge you face may not be food, but the consumption of alcohol. Even healthy, antioxidant-laden red wine can have a negative effect on weight loss since alcohol contains massive amounts of energy.

The EDI of alcohol

Why is it important to index alcohol according to the energy a drink provides? We need to count the extra energy that alcohol contributes to our daily energy intakes, as many studies show that, on average, alcohol accounts for 6 per cent of all the energy we consume. This could mean a difference per day of an extra 1150 kJ of energy for men and 800 kJ for women. Reducing the amount of energy we consume by just these two figures can and will lead to weight loss.

The more alcohol we drink, the more energy we consume. Be honest with yourself, how often do you stop at just one glass?

As the table below shows, the amount of energy that alcohol contains per 100 ml is quite small (mainly because an alcoholic drink contains nearly 90 per cent water). However, it shows how the more beer, wine or spirits you consume, the greater the alcohol content and the more super-loaded your day's energy intake will be.

Alcohol type	Energy Density Index EDI	Energy in 1 glass	Energy in 2 glasses	Energy in 1 standard bottle
light beer	4	159	318	500
heavy beer	22	580	1160	840
white wine	14	406	812	2842
red wine	15	424	848	2968
spirits	19	526	1052	5174

The EDI of alcohol shows us that the alcohol in only one drink fits into the low EDI area. Hence most alcohol is not energy dense if only one drink is consumed. However as we drink more and more the energy density increases, and the energy piles up. A quick comparison shows us the huge difference in energy between the low EDI of light beer, 4, compared to regular-strength beer of 22. A more alcoholic drink such as stout has an EDI of 34, which is quite high, indicating a light beer may be more beneficial for unwinding after work than a full-strength stout. Red and white wine have a low EDI, indicating they too have low amounts of energy in only one glass.

A glass or two with dinner

It is common for people to unwind with a beer or two with dinner, or a glass or two of red wine. Although a glass of wine may be healthy for your heart, we assure you that losing 10 kilograms will be healthier for you.

FOOD	EDI	FAT (grams)	CARBOHYDRATE (grams)	PROTEIN (grams)	ALCOHOL	ENERGY (kJ)
steamed rice	18	0	28	3	0	523
chicken and vegetable stir-fry	30	18	20	27	0	1470
red wine (3 glasses)	15	0	0	0	43.2	1270
ice-cream (150 grams)	32	16	30.3	16	0	1165
Total		34	78.3	46	43.2	4428
energy content		28%	28%	16%	28%	

Alcohol contributes almost 30 per cent of the energy of the meal, or 1270 kJ. Although in total the energy of the meal is not excessively high, it is close to our target of around 6000 kJ for the day for a woman. Without the alcohol, the energy of the meal would be only 3158 kJ, almost half of our 6000 kJ. It would take a woman about 4½ hours after dinner to burn up the alcohol, then a further three hours to get through the fat. During the course of the week this can contribute significantly to the body's ability to burn fat energy.

Dining out

Current indications show that we eat 47 per cent of meals away from home, and this will continue to rise as time goes on. If this figure doesn't apply to you and you cook the majority of meals yourself, congratulate yourself.

Yet many of us deny that we purchase a lot of food away from home. If you leave home in the morning with no food packed, then you will buy food. This has a huge impact on weight gain, and especially fat gain as the more food you eat away from home, the greater the chance it will be of a high energy nature.

So why is consuming meals away from home considered to be potentially dangerous to weight gain? What's wrong with eating out, and what about eating out in moderation? Unfortunately the more food you eat away from home the more energy your food is likely to contain. Seeking value for money we are tempted to choose the largest quantity at the best price. Many people gorge at every meal and, as we saw in Chapter 2, the portion sizes of our meals are larger than ever before. Secondly, if your plate of spaghetti is glistening and shiny, then it contains a fair amount of energy, as this glisten factor is due to fat or oil.

Despite what we may think, hard evidence shows that to make restaurant food taste great chefs use massive amounts of fat, such as butter, lard, ghee, oil or combinations of these. This is extremely consistent with the 'fat tastes great' theory. Have a bowl of pasta that has been immersed in a bit of oil and butter, and compare that to pasta that has no oil added to it. You can taste the difference. The plain pasta is a fair amount 'dryer' in appearance without the glisten, never mind the taste. The majority of main-size servings that we buy contain massive amounts of fat. Below is a summary of the fat content alone of various restaurant foods.

These are for standard size servings (what we should be eating) and for large servings (what we usually eat).

RESTAURANT TYPE	FAT (standard size) (grams)	FAT (large size) (grams)
Chinese	22	45
Thai	32	60
Indian	25	52
Vietnamese	16	29
Lebanese	11	23
Spanish/Mexican	18	40

The difference between average sizes and main sizes is quite large when it comes to fat content. Recall that the more fat you eat, the more energy you consume since fat has 2.25 times the energy of either protein or carbohydrate.

To sum up everything in this book so far, we see a consistent pattern with respect to eating. We choose food because we like the taste. Food that contains a lot of fat tastes great, so we are more inclined to eat more of it. We like to eat a lot of food and pay less money for it. The value-for-money theory suggests that we eat foods with a high EDI as the fat enhances the taste of these foods. Low EDI foods are hardly on a restaurant menu, and hence we don't eat low EDI foods when we dine out.

Weekend eating

Many people tell us that they eat reasonably well during the week but go silly with food and drink on the weekend. You will see that going a little silly can have a huge effect on weight, especially if one manages to slip up a few times with sloppy eating during the week. Also we will analyse the impact here of alcohol and its effects on energy metabolism, as alcohol is one of the pleasures that accompanies restaurant food.

When B Personal analysed the actual energy intakes during a typical night out, we were completely blown away. In our wildest imagination we didn't think people could pack away so much, but you will have to read on to see for yourself. You will also be stunned to see how much energy alcohol contributes to the total energy intake during a night out! If you claim that weight loss is difficult, but can't give up your Saturday night extravaganza with friends, restaurant food could be the source of the problem.

Chelsea's Chinese cravings

Chelsea loves eating Chinese food. In fact when the weekend finally arrives she takes great pleasure in dining out at her favourite Chinese restaurant, with a few drinks and friends. Chelsea is conscious of what she eats as she is trying to lose weight. Her eating and drinking are outlined below, and as you will to see, Chelsea eats a lot of food, although she believes she is just eating normally.

FOOD	EDI	FAT (grams)	CARBOHYDRATE (grams)	PROTEIN (grams)	ALCOHOL	ENERGY (kJ)
2 spring rolls	34	15	45	14	0	1550
pork with plum sauce	38	36	20	27	0	2080
fried rice	29	15	49	10	0	1600
3 gin and tonics & red wine (2 glasses)	15	0	0	0	72	2125
Total		66	114	51	72	7355
energy content		35%	24%	12%	29%	

In one meal Chelsea has eaten over 7000 kJ, more energy than an average woman eats in a single day and certainly more than the recommended target of 6000 kJ. Her 7355 kJ is a whopping amount of energy, but we have to tell you that from our dietary analysis of most restaurant meals consumed by women it's almost an average value. There are no foods that have an EDI value below 10 here, which also is an indicator of a high-energy meal. Many women would call this a moderate meal, but as you can see clearly it isn't.

Under the impression that red wine is good for her, Chelsea uses this as an excuse to drink as much red wine as she wants. How many of us do this, claiming that we're only doing what health authorities recommend, drink red wine! For this meal fat accounts for 66 g or 35 per cent of the total energy intake, carbohydrates 24 per cent and protein 12 per cent. Alcohol has given Chelsea nearly one-third of all her energy for the night. Two large glasses of red wine and 3 gin and tonics is excessive and in terms of energy it contributes almost the same amount of energy as fat does (29 per cent). The sad thing about this lethal combination of alcohol and fat is that they work against each other, competing to be metabolised (see pages 101–107), with alcohol being used as the body's energy source first, fat second.

As we have already shown, alcohol inhibits fat metabolism, and the more alcohol you drink the longer you prevent fat being burnt. Remember also that alcohol has only a little less energy per gram than fat. There is another factor about Chelsea's alcohol consumption that you may find disturbing. How does drinking that much in one night impact on the energy eaten during the total week?

A quick calculation shows that if Chelsea ate 8000 kJ per day, then she would eat 8000 × 7 = 56 000 kJ per week. Four to five glasses of alcohol contain 2125 kJ of energy, which is 3.8 per cent of the energy total that Chelsea eats for the week. If Chelsea manages to sneak in another three to four glasses of red during the week, then she would be taking in 7 per cent of her energy each week from alcohol alone. This is a massive amount of energy, especially if Chelsea is trying to lose weight. This will only hinder her.

How does Chelsea's dinner contribute to her daily energy intake? Her dinner boosts her day's energy intake to around 12 700 kJ. Before dinner she had eaten 5300 kJ (not a great day), and even if she'd taken a little more care and eaten a total of 8000 kJ that day her intake wouldn't have been so bad in terms of energy and weight gain. The amount of 12 700 kJ is horrendously high.

CHELSEA'S CURBED CHINESE CRAVINGS

FOOD	EDI	FAT (grams)	CARBOHYDRATE (grams)	PROTEIN (grams)	ALCOHOL	ENERGY (kJ)
chicken and sweet corn soup (small)	14	8	5	21	0	768
chicken with almonds	21	9	8	20	0	500
steamed rice	18	0	28	3	0	523
red wine (1 glass)	15	0	0	0	14.4	423
Total		17	41	44	14.4	2214
energy content		29%	31%	20%	19%	

Here Chelsea has done a remarkable job reducing the amount of energy she eats when dining at her Chinese restaurant (down by over 5000 kJ). Let's face facts. No one is going to lose weight while eating over 7300 kJ in a single meal. A meal size of 2214 kJ is a much better result for Chelsea. Eating 5000 kJ of food less when she dines out sets her on the right track to lose weight. She cuts her fat down from 66 grams to only 17, her carbohydrate and protein intakes are down from 114 and 51 grams to 41 and 44 grams, respectively; and her alcohol is down from 72 grams (5 glasses) to 14.4 grams found in one drink.

The contribution of alcohol to the total energy of her meal has dropped from 29 per cent to 19 per cent. How was she able to do this? It had a lot to do with the chicken and sweet corn soup, because soup contains plenty of water, hence plenty of volume, and its watery nature reaches or taps receptors that tell the brain to stop eating (see also page 44).

Scientists believe that this could be a key reason why Asian societies are lean – the amount of watery soup dishes they eat. Think about the last time you had soup for an entree and how much food you ate afterwards? Chances are you were able to eat less than usual, as the watery soup triggered this slimming process. The soup has an EDI of 14, which is definitely much lower than 34, the EDI of the spring rolls.

No one is going to lose weight by eating the way Chelsea did the first time around. But weight loss will definitely result from eating low EDI foods as illustrated by her choice of steamed rice, chicken and almonds and only 1 glass of red wine, which have EDIs of 18, 21, and 15 respectively. This is in contrast to her first choice of fried rice, pork in plum sauce and 5 glasses of alcohol, yielding EDI values of 29, 38 and 15 respectively. Using the EDI to choose foods that are lower in energy is an extremely useful weight-loss tool.

Charles' Chinese feast
Charles likes to eat a lot. The feeling of fullness leads mostly to satisfaction and, as our simply dietary analysis shows, Charles has eaten in one meal as much energy as a man usually eats in an entire day. Charles's 10 814 kJ of energy falls just short of the 11 500 kJ of the average man, and makes ups 94 per cent of this energy intake. How on earth is Charles supposed to lose weight when he eats so much food? Where does all this energy come from? Well, 25 per cent of all his energy comes from alcohol.

FOOD	EDI	FAT (grams)	CARBOHYDRATE (grams)	PROTEIN (grams)	ALCOHOL	ENERGY (kJ)
2 spring rolls	34	15	45	14	0	1550
pork with plum sauce	38	36	20	27	0	2150
fried rice	29	20	60	15	0	2016
crispy skin chicken	39	36	10	55	0	2452
beer (6 glasses)	22	0	0	0	90	2646
Total		107	135	111	90	10 814
energy content		37%	21%	17%	25%	

Like Chelsea, Charles has obtained his energy from alcohol and eaten large amounts of fat (a whopping 107 grams). The diet starts Monday, he mumbles. Adding up his total energy for the day shows that he ate 18 500 kJ. This is almost as much food as a marathon runner eats while training for a 42-kilometre run, but Charles, like the majority of men in the Western world, is relatively inactive. 'You have to live and have some fun,' he says, but in reality 18 500 kJ per day and 10 814 kJ in one meal will only lead to weight gain and, if he continues to eat this way, inevitably heart disease or diabetes will follow.

So what can Charles do to curb his eating when he dines out? As the table clearly shows, Charles has eaten food that contains high EDI values. In fact the energy content of these foods is so massively high that most of the foods have an EDI above 30. Charles must include some low EDI foods in here somewhere, preferably right at the beginning. This will provide weight and volume through water, and hence signal to his brain earlier in the meal that his appetite is satisfied.

CHARLES' CURBED CHINESE FEAST

FOOD	EDI	FAT (grams)	CARBOHYDRATE (grams)	PROTEIN (grams)	ALCOHOL	ENERGY (kJ)
Chinese broccoli	1	0.1	1.3	2.5	0	93
beef in black bean sauce	16	14	7	14	0	880
vegetable stir-fry	17	8	8	1	0	470
steamed rice	18	0	28	3	0	523
light beer (2 glasses)	4	0	0	0	5.3	160
Total		22.1	44.3	20.5	5.3	2126
energy content		39%	35%	17%	7%	

Since you are reading this book you must be looking for ways in which to lose weight. And you'll need to do this when you are put to the ultimate test – eating out at a restaurant. As you can see from Charles's new awareness, he manages to use the EDI to recognise which foods contain large amounts of energy that will lead to weight gain and which foods contain lower amounts of energy that will lead to weight loss. This knowledge enables Charles to wipe off a whopping 8688 kJ from his usual restaurant food binge eating.

We cannot help but emphasise what a huge energy saving this is. How is this possible, you may ask, as both meals look remarkably similar? As studies show over and over again, foods that fit the description of being low EDI foods add bulk to any meal. This added bulk means that you feel full on less food. This is found in the Chinese broccoli and stir-fried vegetables. Charles is also able to recognise the differences in EDI of both steamed rice and fried rice.

With the EDI Charles can also see what foods on his menu have low or high values. The beef in black bean sauce had an EDI of only 16, compared to the large EDIs of the others foods such as the crispy skin chicken. Charles manages to choose all of his restaurant dishes from foods that have EDIs of less than 20. The bulkiness of his entrée, and the vegetable stir-fry reduce the amount of food he eats; yet he still feels full with one-fifth the amount of energy. Switching from an excess of full strength beer to a more sensible amount of low alcohol beer also has a huge impact on Charles's energy for the meal. This is superb.

Carmel's Italian passion
The following table describes a typical night out for Carmel who adores Italian cuisine. Unfortunately the energy she consumes is high (nearly 70 per cent of what a typical woman would eat in a day). Comparing her intake to that of Chelsea's 7355kJ in one meal, Carmel has consumed less food and less energy. Yet Carmel would have trouble losing weight this way, especially as we see she is consuming foods that have high EDI values and alcohol still contributes significantly to her energy.

FOOD	EDI	FAT (grams)	CARBOHYDRATE (grams)	PROTEIN (grams)	ALCOHOL	ENERGY (kJ)
fettuccine carbonara entrée	34	20	25	20	0	1500
veal marsala	32	21.2	11.2	39.6	0	1640
gelato	21	0	34	1	0	560
1 vodka and tonic & red wine (2 glasses)	15	0	0	0	32	941
Total		41.2	70.2	60.6	32	4641
energy content		34%	24%	22%	20%	

Carmel's second attempt yields a much better result in her quest to lose weight. She eats only 2193 kJ, which is 50 per cent less than 4641 kJ. She orders the minestrone soup, cutting 1240 kJ from her first entrée choice, which was a fettuccine carbonara made with cream. For her main meal she orders a fettuccine marinara with a tomato base and she requests that the dish be served with no oil. Carmel manages to choose the majority of foods with an EDI value of less than 20. You can see the pattern that is emerging that will undoubtedly help you when dining out.

CARMEL'S IMPROVED EDI MEAL

FOOD	EDI	FAT (grams)	CARBOHYDRATE (grams)	PROTEIN (grams)	ALCOHOL	ENERGY (kJ)
minestrone soup (small)	7	1	9	4	0	260
marinara (tomato based)	20	8	20	18	0	950
gelato	21	0	34	1	0	560
red wine (1 glass)	15	0	0	0	14.4	423
Total		9	63	23	14.4	2193
energy content		16%	48%	18%	19%	

Terry's taste for Thai

During the week Terry is pretty good with his eating, but when the weekend comes around he just has to overindulge. Trying to get Terry to eat well when he goes out is almost out of the question. This is because the feeling of fullness after a meal is something that he has become accustomed to, so he never gives the amount of food he's eaten when dining out a single thought.

FOOD	EDI	FAT (grams)	CARBOHYDRATE (grams)	PROTEIN (grams)	ALCOHOL	ENERGY (kJ)
satay sticks in peanut sauce	32	28	11	46	0	2100
red beef curry	39	26	13	28	0	1630
green chicken curry	20	57	30	66	0	3824
steamed rice	18	0	28	3	0	523
beer (6 large glasses)	22	0	0	0	90	2646
Total		115	82	143	90	10723
energy content		40%	13%	22%	25%	

Unfortunately, Terry has eaten far too much food to induce any kind of weight loss. His fat intake is huge, as Thai main dishes are very high in fat. Like many men, Terry doesn't just eat an average serving; he has some of his wife's green chicken curry and whatever is left uneaten. The interesting thing about the way most men eat is that they are not particularly interested in rice or vegetables. It seems manly to eat meat, and this Terry does, munching on as many chicken and beef dishes as he can. His protein intake in this respect is a whopping 143 grams with only 82 grams of carbohydrate. The 90 grams of alcohol also contributes to his massive 10723 kJ of food eaten, as does the 115 grams of fat.

A DIFFERENT APPROACH FOR TERRY

FOOD	EDI	FAT (grams)	CARBOHYDRATE (grams)	PROTEIN (grams)	ALCOHOL	ENERGY (kJ)
spicy prawn soup	4	3	5	20	0	520
Thai beef salad	14	10	8	40	0	1200
red beef curry with vegetables	26	13	10	14	0	900
steamed rice	18	0	28	3	0	523
light beer (2 glasses)	4	0	0	0	5.3	160
Total		26	51	77	5.3	3303
energy content		30%	26%	39%	5%	

The spicy prawn soup, although not what you would consider to be extremely healthy (compared to the nutritional excellence of minestrone soup), is a far better choice than the first chicken satay sticks covered in energy-dense peanut sauce. Terry has managed to reduce the energy density of his food quite considerably and this will help with his reduction in weight. Like so many men who just cannot control the urge to overeat, Terry battles with weight, blaming one thing or another, but his overeating is the main culprit. Terry still manages to eat his favourite Thai red beef curry, but has done it in a better way. The majority of his meals have an EDI value of less than 20, with the water from the soup and the vegetables adding volume to his food, and hence he reduces the energy density of his night out.

Observing the case studies in this chapter so far clearly

demonstrates that when fat consumption is low, then energy intake is also low. When both fat and alcohol are low the energy consumed is lowered even further. When fat and alcohol are reduced and fibre increased (through eating low EDI foods), the energy a person consumes reduces even further to that of a weight-loss energy intake. Many people looking for the key to weight loss, may find it in the way we eat during the weekend, or whenever eating food away from home.

Isabella's Indian addiction

Isabella loves Indian food, but is also supposedly watching her weight. She has decided to curb the amount she eats, as she knows the more food she eats, the more weight she will gain, especially when it comes to dining out. Isabella is careful about what she eats, but simply loves unwinding with a drink or three.

FOOD	EDI	FAT (grams)	CARBOHYDRATE (grams)	PROTEIN (grams)	ALCOHOL	ENERGY (kJ)
2 samosa	31	18	42	12	0	1600
1 roti	22	7	38	8	0	1168
chicken tikka	29	9	0	25	0	750
potato/pea curry	13	7	6	7	0	340
champagne (2 glasses) & red wine (2 glasses)	15	0	0	0	50	1470
Total		41	80	52	50	5328
energy content		29%	25%	17%	28%	

The eating part of Isabella's Saturday night is very good, as many Indian favourites can be quite fatty and have a lot of energy. She has done well to recognise and avoid these foods. Her choices of chicken tikka and potato and pea curry are reasonably good, and she only consumes small servings of them. Unfortunately her entree is quite energy dense and her alcohol consumption add up to 28 per cent of her total energy for the night.

Her total energy intake for the night is 5328 kJ, which is very large, and will do nothing to aid her quest for weight loss. If she replaces her 4 glasses of alcohol with water, then she would save nearly 1500 kJ. She should aim for an energy intake of about 2000 kJ if she is serious about weight loss, otherwise this extra energy will convert to body fat.

Ivan's Indian indulgence

Ivan does his best not to overeat when he eats out. He is not a drinker, but as you can see, it is sometimes extremely challenging to eat well when dining out. His portion sizes are small, but his energy for the meal still amasses 4618 kJ. Although this is not extreme in terms of what our previous clients have eaten, it may still not be enough to induce a weight change for Ivan. An evening meal of below 3000 kJ is recommended, and he is still over this limit. If Ivan substitutes some vegetable dishes for a chicken dish and some steamed rice for the roti, he will lower considerably the energy density of his meal.

FOOD	EDI	FAT (grams)	CARBOHYDRATE (grams)	PROTEIN (grams)	ALCOHOL	ENERGY (kJ)
1 samosa	31	9	21	6	0	800
1 roti	22	7	38	8	0	1168
chicken tikka (small)	29	9	0	25	0	750
butter chicken (average)	36	38	4	28	0	1900
mineral water (4 glasses)	0	0	0	0	0	0
Total		63	63	67	0	4618
energy content		52%	23%	24%	0%	

Energy Density Index of takeaway foods

All portions are 100 grams unless otherwise stated.

CHINESE FOOD

FOOD	EDI	ENERGY per serve (kJ)
Chinese broccoli	1	71
beef in black bean sauce	16	900
steamed rice (standard serve)	18	993
prawns in satay sauce	20	1200
chicken and almonds	21	1167
pork braised in vegetables	25	1329
chicken chow mien	27	1430
prawn cutlets	27	1500
chicken sweet corn soup	15	780

FOOD	EDI	ENERGY per serve (kJ)
fried rice	29	1520
beef teriyaki	29	1590
prawn omelet	29	1450
beef satay	30	1620
fried noodles	31	1600
lemon chicken	32	1689
spring rolls	34	1700
duck, deep fried with lemon sauce	37	1967
pork in plum sauce	38	2000
crisp skin chicken	39	2004

ITALIAN FOOD

FOOD	EDI	ENERGY per serve (kJ)
minestrone soup	7	450
Siena cake	18	860
chicken cacciatore	19	990
fettuccine marinara (tomato-based)	20	1020
antipasto	21	890
gelato (4 scoops)	21	1050

FOOD	EDI	ENERGY per serve (kJ)
ravioli (200 g)	23	1260
potato gnocchi bolognaise (200 g)	25	1252
cannelloni	25	1420
potato gnocchi	25	1260
pesto (200 g)	26	1326
spaghetti bolognaise	26	1010
¼ pizza supreme	30	1465
osso bucco	32	1726
veal marsala	32	1570
carbonara (200 g)	34	1376
saltimbocca	36	1907
lasagne (200 g)	45	1216
alfredo (large)	46	2361
tortellini (200 g) with cream sauce	54	1760
alfredo	85	2107

THAI FOOD

FOOD	EDI	ENERGY per serve (kJ)
spicy prawn soup (200 g)	4	510
Thai beef salad	14	1287
chicken galangal soup with coconut (200 g)	17	1708
chicken salad	18	1556
green chicken curry (400 g)	20	2329
stir-fry ginger chicken	22	1276
spicy fish cakes (150 g)	26	1040
chicken with basil (300 g)	30	2450
stir-fry prawns with garlic and pepper	31	1474
beef satay with peanut sauce (200 g)	32	1970
beef panang	34	3125
pad Thai (200 g)	34	3482
spring roll	49	1860
mee grob (200 g)	61	3040
curry puffs	70	525

INDIAN FOOD

FOOD	EDI	ENERGY per serve (kJ)
cucumber raita	9	57.4
mulligatawny soup	10	1227
potato pea curry	13	736
dhal lentils	19	1022
steamed rice	19	523
beef vindaloo (200 g)	21	1126
paratha	21	1115
naan bread, 1	22	1201
roti, 1	22	1168
vegetable curry	23	1223
tandoori chicken (200 g)	27	1406
lamb korma	28	1490
chicken tikka (200 g)	29	1540
Kashmiri rice with almonds	29	770
samosas	31	1608
spinach curry	31	1616
butter chicken (200 g)	36	1866
lamb biryani (200 g)	39	1992
pork vindaloo	39	2520
pakora fritters	41	2078
tandoori lamb chops (200 g)	43	2210
meatball curry	43	2184
poppadams	73	473

Summary

People often tell us that they are good during the week and are a little naughty with their eating on the weekend. As you've seen, the role of restaurant food in weight gain is very unproductive! Eating badly on the weekend can result in men consuming 17 000 to 20 000 kJ per day, and women 12 000 to 15 000 kJ. This is more than 100 per cent over what our bodies need and will greatly hinder weight loss. We want you to understand that this is a massive amount of food.

If you find that you are in this situation, and undoubtedly many of us are, you should really eat well and exercise for much of the week to ensure that you get right back on track with your program. But best of all, be vigilant at the restaurant.

- If you are serious about losing weight then cut out alcohol or reduce it to one glass.
- Successful diets limit eating restaurant food to once a week.
- Never dine out when you are extremely hungry.
- Go to our web site and download a copy of these restaurant food EDIs and take them out to dinner with you.
- Include low EDI foods as part of your menu such as soups, vegetables and salads.
- Balance your plate by having more low and moderate EDI foods and less high EDI foods.
- Substitute a dessert at a restaurant with a hot chocolate or flavoured tea.

THE ENERGY DIET AND FAST FOOD

In this chapter you will learn:

- how to get over your guilt
- how to choose better fast food
- why larger portions are letting you down
- the EDI values of fast food

We all eat it!

This book has focused primarily on feeding yourself the right amount of energy to feel alive and energetic, while preventing you from consuming too much of the wrong type of energy that will ultimately result in gaining weight. Eating low EDI foods (better energy foods) more often is at times a challenge. This is especially true when we deal with fast food.

Although we don't really like to admit that we eat much fast food, the reality is that fast food chains are growing at an enormous pace all over the world. In fact, some figures show that a fast food chain opens somewhere in the world every minute. This simply wouldn't happen if there wasn't a demand for this type of food. We can deny that we eat fast food as much as we like, but someone has to be eating enough for fast food chains to show massive yearly profits. How many people are going to consume fast food while trying to lose weight, you may ask. From our evidence, the answer is plenty. And don't forget, pizza is fast food too. If you have children, forget to take your lunch to work, or have a very busy day, then fast food is often a fantastic convenience. Parents often say that feeding their children at a fast food restaurant, where they can relax and eat, is just so convenient. No cooking, no cleaning up, no mess, and, above all, the children are happy.

Fast food guilt

Nobody likes to admit too often that they consume or like to consume fast food on a regular or even semi-regular basis.

As we get older, admitting to consuming fast food regularly sounds incredibly unhealthy. It even sounds cheap and lazy. People fail to admit the frequency with which they consume fast food or takeaway food, especially when they have children, as they fear, we are told, that they will be judged as bad, lazy, irresponsible parents.

The EDI and fast food

The table on the next page shows common fast foods and their accompanying EDI values. As you can see most of the foods you buy at fast food chains have large EDI values. These values are large, indicating they have massive amounts of energy, are not very filling and contain very little in the way of fibre. Remember also that fibre gives you sustained energy, while foods high in fat allow you to eat more and feel full only after lots of food rather than less.

Remember Chapter 3, where we described the filling effects of fibre-containing foods. Well, fast foods are quite the opposite, and as their name suggests these foods can be eaten and digested quickly as the fibre has been removed through processing. Have you ever wondered how a friend can eat two or three hamburgers in one sitting? Have you seen a man boast of eating a family pizza all by himself? Because there's so little fibre and so much fat, the volume of food that can be eaten is massive and the energy consumed even larger. How many bananas could the same person eat? Four maybe five, as the fibre provides the 'stop eating signal' to the brain. Try and make your own homemade hamburgers full of fresh ingredients and you may struggle to eat one.

Fast food servings

The high EDI of fast food isn't the whole problem, however. The volume of food consumed is another drawback, as servings of fast food are massive and force us to overeat, even when we don't feel like it. A full list of fast foods and their accompanying EDI values are listed at the end of this chapter. To give you an idea of how much food and energy typical people may consume during a typical meal of fast food, we have summarised over 200 client dietary analyses of what is commonly eaten.

A TYPICAL SERVING FOR A BIG EATER

FOOD	ENERGY DENSITY (kJ)	FAT (grams)	CARBOHYDRATE (grams)	PROTEIN (grams)	FIBRE (grams)
chicken nuggets (7 pieces)	1533	21.2	20.3	23.3	0.8
large hamburger	3000	48	40	30	2.1
large fries	2100	28.2	54.2	5.4	2.0
large soft drink	912	0	56.5	0	0
Total	7545	97.4	171	58.7	4.9

A typical serving for a big eater reveals the frighteningly large amount of energy consumed from what many consider to be a value-for-money meal. The energy intake of 7545 kJ contributes 66 per cent of the total daily energy consumed by a typical male. For a woman, this meal contributes 94 per cent of her energy needs. Remember a typical man eats about 11 500 kJ and a woman about 8000 kJ.

The amount of fat we eat in a typical day is around 100 grams for men and about 70 grams for women. Consider then the big eater who has eaten 97.4 grams of fat, and polished it off with 171 grams of sugar, which incidentally meets the human requirement for carbohydrates. The 58.7 grams of protein contributes to nearly 80 per cent of the average person's daily protein needs. If you think that it couldn't get any worse, then consider that if you ate this for lunch, then you are unlikely to compensate by having a small dinner. Studies show that after a large serve of fast food, we eat the same amount in our other meals for the day. Does this then mean that people who eat like this even on one day consume 15 200 kJ and 12 800 kJ for men and women respectively? The answer is yes!

ANOTHER TYPICAL SERVING: A REGULAR SERVE

FOOD	ENERGY DENSITY (kJ)	FAT (grams)	CARBOHYDRATE (grams)	PROTEIN (grams)	FIBRE (grams)
chicken nuggets (5 pieces)	1178	16.3	15.6	18	0.6
chicken burger	2144	25	35.4	35.3	2
regular chips	1838	24.6	47.5	5	5
regular soft drink	657	0	40	0	0
Total	5817	65.9	138.5	53.3	7.6

We see here that even a regular-sized serving of fast food is very energy dense, and a single sitting can yield a massive 5817 kJ of energy of which 43 per cent is derived from fat. For those conscious of weight gain and consuming the wrong energy, the 65.9 grams of animal fat and 58.5 grams of sugar are not going to benefit you. An energy intake of 5817 kJ represents 50 per cent of the total energy a male would eat for the day and 73 per cent of what a typical female would eat each day.

Many of us might think that we've done the right thing by choosing the regular size over the large size, and that this amount of food won't be so damaging to our weight-loss cause. But even this meal would force you to eat more energy than your body needs. Ideally, a woman should aim for an energy intake of 6000 kJ for perfect weight loss. this simple high energy meal is 97 per cent of the energy you need. Although some fast food seems harmless enough, if you're trying to lose but have an appetite for fast food, albeit occasionally, it could be one of the reasons you're not losing weight.

ANOTHER TYPICAL SERVING: A SMALL NIBBLE WITH THE KIDS

FOOD	ENERGY DENSITY (kJ)	FAT (grams)	CARBOHYDRATE (grams)	PROTEIN (grams)	FIBRE (grams)
chicken nuggets (4 pieces)	1277	17.7	17	19	0.7
small cheese burger	1754	16.9	43.4	21.7	3
small fries	1181	15.8	30.5	3	3
small orange juice	289	0.2	14.9	1.2	0.6
Total	4501	50.6	106	45	7.3

This scenario is designed to show you that even when we think we are just having a bite to eat, a nibble with the children, or are small eaters, we can still amass 4501 kJ of energy with this fast food snack, which put in perspective is very large. Many people use their children as an excuse to eat fast food, because it is convenient – there's no cooking, mess or washing up. However, convenience will do nothing for your waistline.

This 4501 kJ contributes 40 per cent and 56 per cent of men and woman's daily energy intakes. Remembering that we don't compensate for this later in the day by eating less food, means we could potentially eat 12 200 kJ and 9 825 kJ for men and women respectively, which once again shows gross overeating of energy. How are you going to lose weight by nibbling?

Pizza

Just one slice of pizza contains enough energy to really affect weight gain. Servings of pizza (a slice of pizza is roughly 100 grams) are laden with massive amounts of energy. Their cheesy nature, especially when extra cheese is added, can contribute significantly to the energy you consume. Here is a case study that shows what most of us would consider to be a modest snack. A mere 4 slices of pizza, no extra cheese, can add 5600 kJ to your waistline. Top this off with a soft drink or two and you have over 6257 kJ of energy.

FOOD	ENERGY DENSITY (kJ)
4 slices pizza	5600
regular soft drink	657
Total	6257

Upsizing your waistline even further

If you think that's all there is to fast food, then you're very wrong. Fast food outlets are selling more food to their consumers than ever before. This is true when you consider the value for money a person gets when they upsize their meal. Upsizing is essentially getting better value, or more food for a very small additional cost. You can upgrade a small meal and get a larger one for as little as 50 cents. Some may say that this is a good thing, but stop and think for a moment of the main target audience . . . children. Children, just like adults, are taught that they too can get the value-for-money deals, forcing them to eat more food, even if they don't want to, as it's more economical to purchase more food for less price.

Upsizing doesn't just happen at fast food outlets but anywhere that we purchase food, such as takeaway stalls, and restaurants. The concept of upsizing encourages people, especially children, to consume more energy. It also trains young children and adults that food portion sizes need to be large in order to be satisfying. We know that most fast food restaurants cook in animal fats, as opposed to vegetable fats, and we also know the risks that animal fats play with heart disease.

It must also be stressed that eating fast food once a week, if your diet is low in fat and energy, may not have any deleterious effects, but several times per week due to what people claim is an 'addiction' is a very different story.

A short list of a variety of fast foods follows. A more

comprehensive list of fast foods and their EDIs can be found on our web site: www.bpersonal.com.au. On these lists you will see that the vast majority of fast foods have very high EDIs. Foods such as ice-cream, sundaes and thick shakes have moderately low to moderate EDIs because they are very high in water, and lower in fat and sugar per 100 grams than other fast foods. The surprise food here is soft drinks. Per 100 ml a soft drink contains only 168 kJ of energy, a little less than the energy of an apple. The only problem is that we drink up to 500 ml at a time leading to the consumption of 876 kJ of energy and 54 grams of sugar (3 tablespoons).

THE EDI OF FAST FOODS

EDI	MISCELLANEOUS FAST FOOD
7	soft drinks
19	thick shake
20	sundaes
26	ice-cream
29	hot dog
31	veggie burger
34	vegetarian pizza
35	tacos
36	dim sim
37	spring roll
38	pastie
39	pie
40	large burger

EDI	MISCELLANEOUS FAST FOOD
41	cheese burger
41	bacon and cheese sandwich
41	potato cake
45	chicken burgers
48	sausage roll
49	pizza with the lot
50	chicken nuggets
51	fries
51	nachos
56	hot chips
64	fish and chips

Summary

In the past we have acknowledged that people generally slacken their diets on the weekends and often eat pizza or fish and chips as a treat. Until now we did not realise exactly how much energy these meals contain. With the revolutionary EDI we know now that when we eat large amounts of food containing large amounts of energy, we hinder the process of weight loss, and promote the very opposite – weight gain.

HOW ACTIVE ARE YOU? THE BILSBOROUGH PROGRAM

In this chapter you will learn:

- the importance of the Bilsborough Program for long-term fat loss
- the energy density of typical meals are too great to be overcome by small amounts of exercise
- the best way to exercise to lose weight and for fat loss
- how different exercises burn different amounts of energy
- incidental activity burns small but accumulative amounts of fat and is important for fat loss
- we need to be physically active every day, not just three times a week

How active are you?

Would you classify yourself as an active person? Do you go for a walk or run once or twice a week? Perhaps you go to the gym twice a week? This should be keeping you fit and healthy, you think. You should be losing weight with this kind of exercise. But are you?

With this new concept of energy density we've discovered another very frightening aspect of weight loss. Unfortunately, in today's society physical activity is at an absolute minimum. It isn't considered the 'norm', as 50 to 75 per cent of people *hardly move at all*, and the percentage of inactive people is constantly growing. If there was one component in our lives we could change that would dramatically reduce weight gain, obesity and clear the world of 90 per cent of Western diseases it would be for everyone to be physically active. This doesn't mean just going to the gym three times a week, nor does it mean simply going for a walk three times a week, although these things are certainly a start. Being active means the amount of time you spend on your feet each day.

When you consider that most of us get up in the morning, get in the car, drive to work, sit at a computer all day, drive home, then sit on the sofa and watch TV all night, it's not surprising that we're not losing weight. The problem is that so many of us think that we can balance out this kind of lifestyle by going for a run a couple of times a week and we'll be okay. Wrong!

In this chapter you'll find out how much you need to move around each day and how you can achieve that in order to drop those kilos.

Incidental activity

The first part of being more physically active is to increase every-
day or incidental activity. It's amazing how easy it is to increase
the sheer volume of activity throughout a day without even setting aside a specific time devoted to exercise. Incidental activity
is really low to moderate intensity exercise – the 'exercise you do
when you're not doing exercise'. Look at the list below and check
whether you have done any of these activities recently. If not,
they should be quite easy to include in your day.

INCIDENTAL ACTIVITY	TIME SPENT DOING ACTIVITY	WOMEN – ENERGY USED (kJ)	MEN – ENERGY USED (kJ)
washing dishes	30 minutes	361	420
ironing	1 hour	723	820
mopping floors	45 minutes	1300	1470
making the bed	5 minutes	53	60
mowing the lawn	1 hour	1890	2142
raking leaves	25 minutes	535	600
trimming shrubs	45 minutes	1063	1200
painting	1 hour	1575	1800
playing with children	2 hours	2520	2850
walking up stairs	2 minutes	74	84
walking up stairs five times a day	10 minutes	370	420

Although some daily incidental activity only lasts for several
minutes, and only burns small amounts of energy, when done
every day along with other incidental activity, the amount
of fat used in a day can add up to significant amounts. Take
working around the house or cleaning up, for example. A

weekend of mowing the lawns, trimming shrubs, raking leaves and playing with children can mean from 6000 to 7000 kJ of energy being used. Remember Chelsea and Charles and their huge energy intakes (pages 113 and 117)? Following their bad day with a day spent almost wholly outdoors, expending 6000 to 7000 kJ, is one sure way of balancing the energy they have eaten with exercise.

Getting on your feet

The second way to be more physically active is to increase the number of steps you take each day. You probably don't realise it but if you walk to the train station to catch the train to work instead of just walking to the garage, or if you walk up the stairs instead of catching the lift, or if you walk around to someone else's office rather than calling them, you are increasing your physical activity. This is a very big step forward.

By using a pedometer (a device that measures how many steps people take each day), we can gauge exactly how active or inactive people are. At B Personal we've been working with this concept for some time. What we have found is astonishing. People are hardly moving! For example, Ben, who considers himself quite active, is in fact inactive! How does this come about? Ben runs three times a week – 5 kilometres in about 25 minutes. Does this classify Ben as an active person? Most people would say yes. But on a closer inspection by monitoring his pedometer readings on a daily basis, we found that on the days that Ben isn't running, he isn't really moving around. Like many people who are stuck at a desk or have an inactive job, Ben is taking only 2500 to 3000 steps each day. The equivalent of 1.6 to 1.9 kms. This is classified as very inactive. On the days when Ben runs, he takes about 8000 steps each day. This is a good start, but there is increasing research to suggest that we should all be aiming for 10 000 steps a day.

BEN'S WEEKLY STEPS

Monday	8765
Tuesday	2457
Wednesday	7976
Thursday	3011
Friday	7564
Saturday	3245
Sunday	4678
TOTAL	37696
Average	**5385 steps per day**

Like nearly 90 per cent of people we have analysed, the problem Ben has is because he may go for a walk three times a week, or to the gym, and hence classifies himself as active, his daily routine is so sedentary that he is in fact classified as an inactive person!

This is the greatest revolutionary concept when it comes to weight loss. Exercising three to four times a week needs to be done in the context or against the backdrop of incidental activity. It's the incidental activity that's the most important thing – not the dedicated run or gym session. If you have struggled to lose weight, then there is a rather strong chance that your backdrop of incidental activity is very low, and probably much lower than you might credit. Combine increased activity with a low EDI diet and we promise you that you will see the weight fall away.

Recently I was speaking at a hospital to overweight and obese patients. One woman who had lost 45 kilograms told me that she started increasing her incidental activity, simply by walking to her letterbox and back each day. Then she progressed to walking to the milk bar to get the paper on a daily basis. She gradually increased her step count from as little as 1000 each day.

It is from this earth-shattering data that we have come to devise **The Bilsborough Program**. We can guarantee that by following this program you will not only get lean, but stay lean. This is a big promise, but when you see the 'no gimmicks' program rolled out in front of you, you'll see why it is so successful.

The Bilsborough Program

The Bilsborough Program is based on the relationship between daily steps taken and the energy that these steps burn. For example, it has been estimated that 2500 steps takes about 20 minutes to walk, is the equivalent of 1.6 kilometres (1 mile) and burns up about 420 kJ. There are all sorts of factors that can affect these calculations, but these figures are a very good approximate. The main construct of the Bilsborough Program is to first identify where you are exactly when it comes to your daily physical activity. For many of our clients who have undergone this initial analysis (Stage 1), their reaction has been shock. From here we progress to gradually increase the number of steps we take each week, and hence the amount of energy we burn. We then stabilise before increasing our step count and energy expenditure even further.

Stage 1 *Initial analysis*

You need to establish exactly how physically active you are. Stage 1 involves you recording a week's worth of steps from Monday to Sunday. (The following is a record of a client of ours.)

CATHERINE

DAY	STEPS	ENERGY BURNT (kJ) (2500 STEPS = 420 kJ)	km
Monday	2346	394	1.5
Tuesday	2256	379	1.4
Wednesday	4567	767	2.9
Thursday	2378	399	1.5
Friday	2089	351	1.3
Saturday	1987	334	1.2
Sunday	3986	670	2.5
TOTAL	19 609	3294	12.3 km
Average	2801 steps/ day	470 kJ/day	1.8 km/day

(Once you have the number of steps you can also work out how many kJ you've burned and also how many kilometres you've covered, but this is not necessary. Remember each 2500 steps = 420 kJ or 1.6 km.)

Stage 1 for Catherine clearly defines why she hasn't been losing any weight, despite following a sensible diet. Her active days consist of 35 minutes of walking two days a week, resulting in 4567 steps (Wednesday), and 3986 steps (Sunday). Catherine does consider herself to be active, yet as the pedometer reading clearly shows, most of her days are extremely inactive. The scary thing is that many scientists would consider this to be *gross inactivity*.

When we ask Catherine about her daily movements we learn that she essentially gets out of bed, gets ready for work, walks to the car, sits down at the office, walks back to the car, cooks a quick meal at home and then remains on the couch until bedtime. She burns a mere 470 kJ each day (the energy found in a large apple) and covers a total average daily distance of only 1.8 km. When you consider that our caveman ancestors covered up to 19 km daily, Catherine walks only 9.5 per cent as far daily as her caveman ancestors, and is wondering why she can't lose weight!

When we are first approached by Steve to help manage his weight he weighs about 108 kg. Like many people that we have featured in this book, Steve thinks that he is generally an active person, as he walks the dog for 20 minutes each day and has a pretty busy job. As his week 1 step count shows, he is a reasonably active person, especially compared to Catherine. His daily step count ranges from a low of 5678 steps to a high of 12744 steps. His average daily step count is near the 10000 mark. This step profile is better than Stage 3 (which requires a person to take 5000 steps each day and on two days to take 7000 steps). Steve's step profile, however, is not a consistent model of Stage 4 (which requires a minimum of 8000 steps each day and 12000 steps on two days).

STEVE

DAY	STEPS	ENERGY BURNT (kJ)	km
Monday	5678	954	4
Tuesday	7865	1321	5
Wednesday	9874	1659	6
Thursday	12744	2141	8
Friday	5780	971	4
Saturday	8745	1469	6
Sunday	7699	1293	5
TOTAL	58385	9808	37.38
Average	8341 steps/day	1401 kJ/day	5 km/day

With these results, Steve can bypass Stages 2 and 3 and work on a consistent step profile that matches or betters Stage 4.

Stage 2 **Add 1500 steps**

Increase each day's step count by 1500 steps. (If you feel you can increase your step count even further, then you can go directly to Stages 3, 4, or 5. Our advice for people just starting off, though, is to see through Stage 2.) Stay at Stage 2 until you can achieve an extra 1500 steps consistently each day. For some people, this may take one week, while for others it may take several. That's fine, it's important to go at your own pace.

Increasing your step count by 1500 steps increases the amount of energy you expend each day by 252 kJ. This may not seem like much, but we can assure you that plenty of clients have lost significant weight at Stage 2.

CATHERINE

DAY	STAGE 1 STEPS	STAGE 2 STEPS	ENERGY BURNT (kJ)	km
Monday	2346	3846	646	2.5
Tuesday	2256	3756	631	2.4
Wednesday	4567	6067	1019	3.9
Thursday	2378	3878	1042	3.9
Friday	2089	3589	603	2.3
Saturday	1987	3487	586	2.2
Sunday	3986	5486	921	3.5
TOTAL	19 609	30 109	5448	20.7 km
Average	2801	4301	778	3 km

In Stage 2 on the Bilsborough Program Catherine increases her daily step count by 1500 steps as instructed. To do this Catherine takes more steps during the day at work, and includes incidental activities such as getting out of the office at lunch time, and making a concerted effort to get off her chair at work. All these little steps contribute to the energy she burns up each day. It is these little steps that we think account for nothing, but when strung together make a huge difference.

Catherine's total weekly steps rise from a Stage 1 total of 19 609 to 30 109 steps. This is significant. What is even more significant is the increase in energy expenditure during the two weeks. By taking as little as 1500 extra steps each day, which may take only 10 to 15 minutes of your time, the amount of daily energy expenditure increases from 470 kJ to 778 kJ. This means that Catherine's body is burning more energy each day, which will definitely contribute to either curbing her weight gain, furthering her weight loss, or maintaining the weight she has already lost. Catherine increases her backdrop of incidental activity by over 50 per cent, or from an average of 2801 steps to 4301 each day.

If you have found achieving 1500 extra steps each day challenging, then you should stay on Stage 2 until you can achieve this comfortably. When you have found this achievable, it is time to progress to Stage 3.

Stage 3 5000–7000 steps

Stage 3 involves taking a minimum of 5000 steps each day, and on two days of the week 7000 steps. (If you have already achieved this, go to Stage 4 or 5.) You need to stay on this stage until you can comfortably complete the minimum steps. We have found on average this takes four weeks.

For some people Stage 3 may take some getting used to, especially if you have been classifying yourself as active, but in reality have been taking very few daily steps similar to Catherine. Taking a minimum of 5000 steps each day guarantees that you will expend 840 kJ each day and on two days of the week about 1200 kJ. It may be no surprise to you that we have observed some astonishing weight-loss results at Stage 3.

CATHERINE

DAY	STAGE 3 STEPS	ENERGY BURNT (kJ)	km
Monday	5000	840	3.2
Tuesday	5000	840	3.2
Wednesday	7000	1176	4.5
Thursday	5000	840	3.2
Friday	5000	840	3.2
Saturday	5000	840	3.2
Sunday	7000	1176	4.5
TOTAL	39 000	6552	25 km
Average	5571 steps/day	936 kJ/day	3.5 km/day

Catherine consolidates her backdrop of physical activity at Stage 3 to a daily minimum of 5000 steps. Catherine burns on average 936 kJ of energy every day. This is nearly 100 per cent more energy than she did in stage 1. She has evaluated where she was with her activity output in Stage 1, and then has added little bits of activity to her daily lifestyle.

Stage 4 *Walking to your ideal weight: 8000–12 000 steps*

If you have made it to Stage 4, then you have done very well. You should have noticed some weight change. For some this weight change will be massive. Stage 4 consists of taking a background of 8000 steps each day, with two days a week of 12 000 steps. You need to stay on Stage 4 until you have achieved these minimum steps. It can take up to four weeks to achieve this, but you'll notice the weight dropping off again. You may then opt to stay at this stage to maintain your weight, but for further weight loss go to Stage 5. For some people this stage is sufficient to promote weight loss, and prevent weight gain. It is difficult to develop general rules that will apply to all people, so for some who have started like Catherine and were truly inactive, Stage 4 may be the upper limit.

For anyone currently at Stage 4 or successfully navigating their way through this challenging stage (and eating a diet consisting of low EDI foods), then you are achieving something that is having a huge impact on your metabolism.

CATHERINE

DAY	STAGE 4 STEPS	ENERGY BURNT (kJ)	km
Monday	8000	1344	5.2
Tuesday	8000	1344	5.2
Wednesday	12000	2016	7.7
Thursday	8000	1344	5.2
Friday	8000	1344	5.2
Saturday	8000	1344	5.2
Sunday	12000	2016	7.7
TOTAL	64000	10752	41.4 km
Average	9143 steps/day	1536 kJ/day	6 km/day

Catherine stays at Stage 4 for over eight weeks, until she can consistently do 8000 steps each day. Her daily step count increases to an average of 9143 steps each day. The amount of energy she expends each day rises from a weight gaining 470 kJ, to 1536 kJ or a whopping 227 per cent. Catherine readjusts her lifestyle so that she exercises and achieves her backdrop of physical activity for her 12000 steps each day. On her 8000 step days she does the following:

- walks at lunch time to get lunch   3000 steps
- takes the stairs at work   2400 steps
- walks to the train station and back   2600 steps

STEVE

DAY	WEEK 1 STEPS	ENERGY BURNT (kJ)	km
Monday	8023	1348	5
Tuesday	8110	1362	5
Wednesday	9874	1659	6
Thursday	8224	1382	5
Friday	8001	1344	5
Saturday	12098	2032	8
Sunday	12207	2051	8
TOTAL	66537	11178	42
Average	9505 steps/day	1597 kJ/day	6 km/day

Developing a consistent step profile at Stage 4 is not as easy as Steve first thought. Although he wanted to leap straight into Stage 5, anyone can go out of their way and barnstorm for a week on Stage 5, but that's not what the Bilsborough Program is about. The focus of the program is maintenance over the long term. So though you may feel that you can clock the program this week, or next month, can you maintain Stage 5 for one to two years? Start small and build up. Like Steve, learn that walking to buy the paper each morning gives you a certain number of steps, or that walking once round his neighbourhood block gives him 3000 steps. This way you develop little mental triggers that can help you sustain the program.

Stage 4 for Steve is all about developing consistency, and also learning what has to be done to achieve 12 000 steps. He finds a game of golf (9 holes), two walks around the block, and some housework give him his 12 000 steps. For other people this may mean going for a 40 minute walk/run before you launch into a weight training session (as well as other activities during the day), or simply getting off your backside and onto your feet.

If you have a closer look at Steve's profile, you may notice that he has just managed to scrape in to 8000, and 12 000 steps on his required days. This is not sufficient to progress to Stage 5, as 10 000 steps each day is a considerable but attainable jump from 8000 steps. We want Steve to comfortably reach his Stage 4 targets, not just scrape in, so he will stay at Stage 4 for the time being.

STEVE

DAY	WEEK 12 STEPS	ENERGY BURNT (kJ)	km
Monday	10 287	1728	7
Tuesday	10 087	1695	6
Wednesday	11 267	1893	7
Thursday	11 876	1995	8
Friday	10 236	1720	7
Saturday	10 345	1738	7
Sunday	16 523	2776	11
TOTAL	80 621	13 545	53
Average	11 517 steps/day	1935 kJ/day	7 km/day

After 12 weeks on Stage 4 Steve makes the move to Stage 5. As his profile shows he has consistently cracked the 10000-step mark. His 18 holes of golf on Saturdays and long beach walks on Sundays help with his 15000-step challenge. Other strategies he uses during the week are walking to a park in the city near where he works to eat his lunch (low-to-moderate EDI food), which gives him an extra 2900 steps each day. If he is unable to do this, he has worked out that if he walks the stairs (up and down) a total of four times a day he acquires a further 2400 steps. Two laps at his local park also give him 2500 steps. From the start of his program he has increased the amount of energy his body uses (especially fat energy), by a massive 47% each day.

Stage 5 *10000–20000 steps*

Stage 5 requires a daily step count of 10000 steps and two days of 15000 to 20000 steps. For many people 10000 steps is a real challenge as it requires some serious planning. This stage may appeal to fit people who want to get fitter, or if you're trying to lose those extra few kilograms. You can also spend one to two weeks at this stage and then move back down to Stage 4. We recommend you stay at Stage 4 or 5, if you want to maintain permanent weight loss.

Some people may have found the inspiration to jump straight to Stage 5, while for some people Stage 4 is sufficient to reach their goals. The only way to achieve 15000 to 20000 steps is to stay on your feet for about two hours. On our own

15 000 to 20 000-step day, we aim to get out for a walk for about two to three hours, usually on the weekend. This can be a real challenge and if you can't see yourself doing this, then wash your car, sweep your house, do some gardening, walk to the park with your kids, or play a game of golf. One client found himself walking up and down his corridor at night just to get his pedometer over that 20,000-step challenge. If you have achieved Stage 5 status then you need never look back. For Catherine, maintaining Stage 4 sees her weight plummet 23 kg in 16 weeks.

STEVE

DAY	WEEK 3 STEPS	ENERGY BURNT kJ	km
Monday	11 235	1888	7.2
Tuesday	10 236	1720	6.6
Wednesday	13 529	2273	8.7
Thursday	13 987	2350	9.0
Friday	10 870	1826	6.9
Saturday	20 983	3525	13.5
Sunday	24 812	4168	15.9
TOTAL	105 652	17 750	68 km
Average	15 093 steps/day	2535 kJ/day	9.7 km/day

Steve now walks 105 652 steps each week, covering over 68 km (or 9.7 km a day). The long term sees Steve follow a combination of two weeks of Stage 4 and two weeks of Stage 5 each month. On some of his weekend days he consistently tops the 20 000-step mark, which is a real achievement. His weight plummets from 108 kg to 81 kg in six months, by combining the Bilsborough Program and the Energy Diet. What Steve shows us is that daily incidental activity and a diet lower in energy together give the most potent stimulator of weight loss, especially fat loss.

For some people it may be practical to stay at Stage 5. Dropping back to either Stage 4, or even 3, may be needed during busy times.

How you can do it

The key to losing weight is to have a sufficient backdrop of incidental activity, whether you exercise three to four times a week or not. It is a common mistake for people to call themselves active, when they mistakenly substitute their three walks/runs a week for incidental activity. You cannot lose weight this way, as incidental activity, especially during Stage 5, would add up to more energy used up in a week than the total of your three exercise sessions. The Bilsborough Program is very simple, practical, and should form the basis for any physical activity program. The added cost of a pedometer, can work out to 28 cents a day.

Set yourself a challenge to see what your own record step count can reach. We do this with clients, family and even between ourselves. Our client record at B Personal so far is 47 445 steps. This client, who had typically spent Sundays in front of the TV, now goes for a long walk, plays a game of basketball, plus engaging in other incidental activity. What an effort, yet it is also healthy, competitive and fun.

The Bilsborough Program is not designed to be complicated. It is a very simple, inexpensive program that can be undertaken by anyone at any time. Some weight-loss programs add up to hundreds of dollars. There are no joining fees or huge costs, except a pedometer (costing $20 or less). We know that no matter what level of physical activity you are at, the backdrop of incidental physical activity has to be achieved for consistent and sustainable weight loss.

Some hints for achieving physical activity goals

- Watch less TV.
- Give yourself a maximum of the half-hour news and one program to watch three nights of the week.
- Make it a point to spend more time outdoors.
- Increase the amount of incidental activity you do.
- Make it a goal to do some kind of physical activity each day even if it's weeding the garden.
- Get out and play with your children.
- Make it a goal to find at least 60 minutes a day to be physically active.
- Use your weekends wisely and hire some bikes, go for a long walk or even learn to rollerblade.

- If you are spending your life either in front of a computer or TV you are wasting your life away.
- Spend more times with friends who value fitness as they will encourage you. Unfit people generally won't.
- Do a yoga class once a week to look after your mind and reduce stress.
- Change your expectations: that one-hour of physical activity is not a lot for burning energy! For example, go for a three-hour cycle, or be active for longer than an hour a few times a week.

Summary

We showed you in earlier chapters how to make 'subtle changes' to your food to 'subtly' reduce the amount of energy you eat. In other words the EDI can save you from eating excess energy. Now you need to make subtle changes to your activity levels. If you have struggled to lose weight then you need a 'measure' of your daily activity or inactivity. Try the Bilsborough Program.

THE BEST EXERCISE FOR WEIGHT LOSS

In this chapter you will learn

- how much energy different exercises burn
- how much carbohydrate and fat are burnt with different exercises
- a good exercise program needs to be complemented with a good eating program
- exercising while eating too much energy will not lead to weight loss and can be a key reason why you have tried to lose weight and failed

Sticking with it

Don't be one of those people who gives up before your body has been given a chance to fully reap the benefits of low-intensity exercise! We know that if you persist with low-to-moderate intensity exercise your body will *adapt* so that it is burning fat most effectively. These adaptations are essential to keep your body in energy balance. If you are one of the people who has been doing everything right but still cannot lose weight, then you owe it to yourself to lift your incidental activity. As we have pointed out, you might classify yourself as active because you exercise for three hours of the week. But for the remaining 165 hours in the week what are you doing?

In this chapter we look at all sorts of exercise and assess the best one for *you* – to ensure that you are assisting your weight loss. However, the most important point to remember is that the activities included here will not help you to lose weight significantly if that is all you are doing. They must be combined with a solid background of incidental activity, as described in Chapter 7.

Burning energy through exercise

During a typical day an average *inactive* man's body will burn 9500 kJ of energy, while an average *inactive* woman's body will burn 6500 kJ. This is without physical activity and simply goes towards maintaining a person's metabolism (body heat, breathing, organ function, etc.). By doing physical activity a person then adds to this basic energy expenditure.

For example, one day on the Bilsborough Program at Stage 4 (see page 154) can help your body burn a further 1344 kJ of energy. It is important to keep this in mind when investigating how structured physical activity can add to the burning of energy.

By now you have a good understanding of how the energy in food affects your weight. When you are physically active you have an opportunity to remove some of this excess stored energy by burning or metabolising it. Excess energy is stored as fat. It is critical that you understand that the metabolism of each macronutrient – carbohydrate, protein and fat – is very different, and cannot be treated equally when it comes to simply burning energy.

After the consumption of a hamburger, for example (which contains 2200 kJ of energy, 29 grams of protein, 22 grams of fat and 48 grams of carbohydrate), the speed at which these food components are metabolised is vastly different. First, the protein from the burger will be broken down at a rate of about 6 grams every hour, meaning that all the protein from the burger will be metabolised in five hours. The fat will take about three hours just to get to your bloodstream, and then it will be absorbed at 12 to 15 grams per hour, taking a total of five hours to be metabolised. So the metabolism of fat and protein, in this case, will be roughly the same. On the other hand, 48 grams of carbohydrate will be metabolised in just over an hour. Due to the speed at which carbohydrates are metabolised (and therefore ready to be used by the body), energy from carbohydrate is much easier for the body to access than energy from fat. (This is another reason why low-carbohydrate diets are not well founded – carbohydrates are the easiest thing to burn off!) In order to lose weight efficiently and permanently, you need to exercise at a level that burns fat rather than carbohydrates.

For many people who want to lose a few kilos, the best activity (as well as the most sustainable) is walking or cycling, at a low to moderate intensity.

Burn fat, not carbohydrate

The most common form of physical activity that people undertake in a bid to offset their energy density is aerobic activity. This might be walking, light jogging, cycling, swimming and other fun activities such as team sports and rollerblading. Aerobic exercise is best for permanent weight loss because it burns energy from fat, rather than carbohydrates. During the course of any exercise there are only two fuels that contribute to energy – fat and glucose (glucose comes from carbohydrate). There are many factors that need to be considered in order to use such large amounts of energy from fat and relatively small amounts of glucose.

First, there needs to be plenty of oxygen present if you are going to use the majority of fat from your fat stores (or from your body fat). This means that when you are exercising you shouldn't be out of breath and you should still be able to have a conversation. Fat needs oxygen for it to be released from fat cells during exercise. (For one molecule of fat to be burnt you need 23 molecules of oxygen.) Without oxygen it just remains imprisoned in the fat cells. Take sprinting for the train or bus. When your legs get so heavy they could drop off, and you're left puffing, this is a clear example of not using your fat stores. But in times of oxygen abundance, such as during low to moderate intensity walking, fat can ooze out of the fat cell and drift to the exercising muscles. This drifting process is just that, a slow process, and fat delivery to the muscle cells takes around 15 minutes after the commencement of exercise and can last for many hours. The longer we walk, the more fat our bodies can burn. Incidental activity is also low intensity, and sometimes moderate in nature, which makes it ideal as aerobic and hence fat-burning.

Consider a marathon runner who burns 110 grams of fat and 475 grams of carbohydrates. During a two-hour-plus marathon, the ratio of fat to carbohydrate being used is about 1 to 5. In other words for every 1 gram of fat the body metabolises, 5 grams of carbohydrate are used. But what happens when we exercise longer? On the Tour de France, a daily eight-hour cycle can use 475 grams of fat and about 1100 grams of glucose, or a ratio of 1 gram of fat for every 2 grams of glucose. One reason for this is that the body tries to hold back carbohydrates to be used as a key fuel for the brain, nervous system and the heart, but as time wears on during exercise, this holding back of carbohydrate results in your muscles using less carbohydrate and more fat as fuel. This is why going for a long walk or cycle can result in a greater amount of fat energy being used, and smaller amounts of carbohydrate energy, than happen during jogging or running.

Exercise and appetite suppression

One of the benefits of exercise is that it can suppress the feeling of hunger, especially high intensity vigorous activities. Many people experience a lack of hunger when they complete exercise. The reasons for this are not clearly understood but it seems that exercise may affect the appetite signals to the brain by somehow suppressing them, or telling the brain that you are not hungry. The feeling of not wanting to eat is a common feeling that some people get, especially when the exercise has been strenuous. The other theory is that exercise simply burns energy and this burning of energy decreases our drive to eat. There are studies, however, that show as people get fitter and put on more muscle, they may feel hungrier. This is where it is important to understand that there is no use feeding this hunger with high energy density food, and therefore stacking up on the energy you just expended during your walk. In fact, if you are not prepared with your meals and you are tired and hungry after exercise, there is a real danger that you will lash out and look for a high energy dense snack. Don't undo all of your good work!

Adapting to fitness

When people do moderate-intensity aerobic training, such as a good power walk, they are using specific areas of their muscles. Muscles are comprised of muscle fibres (small bundles of muscle). There are many types of muscle fibres and when you do aerobic training such as power walking, jogging or cycling; your body uses fibre type 1 – 'slow twitch muscle fibres'. These slow twitch muscles fibres are fat-burning fibres, and are responsible for taking up fat and burning it during your power walk. The more you walk, and the fitter you become, the more fat energy these muscles burn. This may take a little time, but if you give your aerobic exercise program some time, this will happen. How do these muscles increase the amount of fat you can burn? These muscle fibres change, adapt and then evolve, so that you can go from being an inactive TV watcher, to an active Stage 4 or 5 fat-burning person. Over time and with consistent, regular aerobic exercise, there will be certain benefits:

- increased general fitness
- increased ability of the body to use more energy
- more blood pumped around the body with each heartbeat
- more oxygen contained in the blood, resulting in more haemoglobin in the blood (good for heart health)
- ability to walk, run or cycle faster without getting tired or having that feeling of leg heaviness.

Let's now use this information to investigate how different activities compare to one another.

How different modes of exercise burn different amounts of energy

This book has focused on why we have trouble losing weight and it is clear that our understanding of energy balance is severely lacking. In Western society we have failed to understand what it takes physically to balance the energy from the food we eat.

In Chapter 5 we observed how Chelsea and Charles typically overconsumed both food and alcohol at dinner. Chelsea consumed 7355 kJ of energy and Charles ate 10 814 kJ in a single meal. For the day they amassed 12 800 kJ and 18 500 kJ, respectively. It is important to understand that this energy intake grossly exceeds what the human body needs during a typical day, yet almost *everyone* overconsumes without knowing it. As we mentioned earlier, the average *inactive* man metabolises 9500 kJ of energy, while the average *inactive* woman's body will burn 6500 kJ. Comparing this to how much energy Chelsea and Charles have eaten, we find that they have eaten an extra 6300 kJ and 9500 kJ, respectively. This sort of eating pattern could well account for 60 to 65 per cent of the world's Western population being either overweight or obese.

Chelsea and Charles want to know what happens to this energy if they exercise the next day. They (wrongly) think that a little exercise the day after a big night brings about a balance. Assuming their feast took place on a Saturday night, we might expect to find them trying to 'burn' it off on the Sunday. How does the body respond to such a large meal and what effects of exercise, if any, will aid in Chelsea and Charles losing weight?

CHELSEA

	FAT (grams)	CARBOHYDRATE (grams)	PROTEIN (grams)	ALCOHOL	ENERGY (kJ)
Total	66	114	51	72	7355

CHARLES

	FAT (grams)	CARBOHYDRATE (grams)	PROTEIN (grams)	ALCOHOL	ENERGY (kJ)
Total	107	135	111	90	10814

An early morning swim or walk

Many people opt for a morning walk or a swim in a bid to lose weight. In *The Fat-Stripping Diet* we showed why swimming is not an optimal exercise for fat loss, but nevertheless can result in the body using significant amounts of energy. The majority of scientific evidence shows that swimming, cycling and running use the same amount of energy, although swimming uses more carbohydrate and less fat than either running or cycling. One solid hour of swimming will burn a significant amount of energy, as the table on the next page shows. However the energy used barely makes a dent in the energy Chelsea and Charles ate and drank at the Chinese restaurant the night before.

The situation is similar for walking, except the energy that the body burns from fat is significantly greater, and the amount from carbohydrate is less. An important factor to consider in favour of walking is that not too many people would be able to swim continuously for an hour. Bearing this in mind, we have adjusted the amount of energy expended during swimming to allow Chelsea and Charles to make several stops. For a very fit person, both of these activities would use more energy.

A 1-HOUR WALK OR SWIM

		ENERGY (kJ)	CARBOHYDRATE (grams)	FAT (grams)
Chelsea	walk	1740	46	25
	swim	1733	62	18
Charles	walk	1970	53	29
	swim	1970	70	22

Is walking better than jogging?
This is one of the most common questions that we get asked. Is it better for a person trying to lose weight to run rather than walk? In fact some people have even gone so far as to say walking is useless, and running burns much more energy and hence much more fat. In recent surveys, including our own web site, 99 per cent of people say they wouldn't or couldn't run to lose weight, but they would be prepared to walk. Another thing that counts against running is the impact pressure on joints and the spine, as well as the risk to the heart of an overweight person unused to running. For how long could an unfit person really run?

When you walk you burn energy; and the faster you walk, the more energy you burn. The faster you walk, the more awkward it feels. Have you ever tried to walk as fast as you can without running? It feels uncoordinated, your hands move around everywhere and your legs stretch out, wanting to bend and start running. You are 'all over the place' with your style and consequently exercising very inefficiently. But this inefficiency means you will burn plenty of energy. It's like driving a car with the doors wide open. Your car will burn more petrol because the added air resistance, provided by the open doors, decreases the efficiency.

If we compare both walking and jogging, we see that at 8 km/hr walking and running burn the same amount of energy. Walking faster means you become less efficient, and hence burn more energy. However, and here is an amazing fact, jogging faster increases efficiency, resulting in a *decreased* amount of energy being spent. Of course, if you broke into a sprint this situation would change and you would burn much more energy.

Many people argue that if you run faster, then you burn more energy, and hence more fat overall. But ask yourself the question, if you are not an elite athlete, how long can you run fast for? How many people can run for as long as they can walk? For fit, well-trained people running is certainly better than walking, but for non-elite people don't underestimate the fat-burning capacity of walking. For someone who is inactive and wants to get fit, or for someone who is just moderately fit, walking is the best exercise. If you are looking for a great fat-loss exercise, you can't go past a good walk.

There are other advantages of walking over jogging.

- Running hurts! Especially for unfit people.
- Walking is something that everyone has access to, unlike gyms, pools and exercise equipment.
- It is easier to get motivated to walk than to run.
- Sticking to a physical activity program based on walking is easier than one based on running.
- Many people hate jogging and will be put off excersing altogether if they are told they must go out and jog.
- Walking is more practical – and much safer! – for unfit people. (Running can be dangerous in terms of heart disease/high blood pressure, etc.)

2–HOUR BIKE RIDE

	ENERGY (kJ)	CARBOHYDRATE (grams)	FAT (grams)
Chelsea	2847	74	37
Charles	4209	126	47

Cycling at low to moderate intensity is an efficient way of burning energy, especially fat energy. A two-hour cycle can contribute significantly to burning off the previous day's food – but only if the food consumed was generally low in energy density. Although individual results vary, the energy breakdown shown here serves as a good approximation of what average people are likely to burn on a bike ride. Most people feel that if they cycle at a good pace for two hours it will be extremely rewarding and they will burn off an extravagant meal eaten the night before.

Unfortunately, this simply is not the case. Chelsea burns a good 2847 kJ or 38 per cent of her evening meal. Her two hours of cycling burns 37 grams of fat (only 56 per cent of her intake) and 74 grams of carbohydrate (65 per cent of her intake). Charles burns 4209 kJ, or 39 per cent of his meal, 47 grams of fat and 126 grams of carbohydrate. Charles is able to burn more carbohydrate and fat than Chelsea as he has more muscle on his body and hence more sites to burn energy. Both use very little protein, which is normal, as the body doesn't use significant amounts of protein during exercise. Cycling burns 1411 kJ per hour for women (and only 36 grams of carbohydrate, and 19 grams of fat) and 2100 kJ for men (with 63 grams carbohydrate and 23.5 grams for men). To have cycled off their meals, Chelsea and Charles would have to cycle for over five hours each! So, eating energy dense meals and then thinking we can exercise it off is a false assumption!

In the above example although Chelsea burnt less fat than Charles, she actually burnt a greater relative amount of fat. One of the more recent breakthroughs in exercise physiology shows that when men and women are matched for fitness and body composition, women can actually burn a greater percentage of energy from fat than men. This means that women burn 50.9 per cent of their energy from fat, while men burn 43.7 per cent. This is great news for women and exercise, as it shows although women are more efficient at storing fat, for the first time we know they are actually better also at losing body fat.

Weight training

What impact would weight training have in terms of energy balance for both Chelsea and Charles? There are many types of resistance-training methods, but here we will focus on the two most common: a circuit-type session where people generally go from one piece of equipment to the next with about a 15-second break between exercises; and a typical weight-training session where a moderate to heavy weight is lifted 8 to 12 times, followed by a rest period usually of a minute, sometimes more. Weight training can be an effective way to lose and maintain weight loss, especially if the energy we eat from food is not high.

WEIGHT TRAINING – MEDIUM INTENSITY

	ENERGY (kJ)	CARBOHYDRATE (grams)	FAT (grams)	PROTEIN (grams)
Chelsea	1150	54	6	0
Charles	1700	80	9	0

Unfortunately for both Chelsea and Charles their one hour of circuit training, although magnificent for their hearts as well as for building some muscle, has barely any impact on their dinner. Chelsea has burnt only 1150 kJ, which is a small fraction of her dinner (~16 per cent), and Charles 1700 kJ (also ~16 per cent). The training intensity that they undertook was of moderate to high intensity. At higher intensities of training the body uses a greater portion of carbohydrate to fat, and this example shows that for every gram of fat being used during circuit-type training, the human body can burn 9 grams of glucose.

WEIGHT TRAINING – HIGH INTENSITY

	ENERGY (kJ)	CARBOHYDRATE (grams)	FAT (grams)	PROTEIN (grams)
Chelsea	1260	60	7	0
Charles	1930	92	10	0

With this type of weight training you usually lift a heavier weight than in the medium-intensity-style circuit. You expend more energy, but you also have a longer rest between sets for recovery. You may lift for 30 minutes and rest for 30 minutes in a typical one hour training session. For our purposes we will assume that both Chelsea and Charles train for 40 minutes and rest for 20 minutes during their hour-long training session. Although they both burn more energy primarily from carbohydrate and not fat, the extra energy they burn is not enough to compensate for the high energy dinner.

A simple calculation shows that if Chelsea and Charles kept this high-intensity training up for about six hours they would burn off their dinner, however it is not physically possible to perform high-intensity activity for longer than 45 minutes to an hour, let alone six hours. Within this 45 minute period you will have to stop, get your breath back, and let the heaviness (lactic acid) clear from the particular muscles you are using.

How many people walk away from their training session believing that they burnt the energy equivalent to that of half a marathon, just because their arms feel good, or their legs are still hurting (in a good way) from doing weights? As we have seen, eating a high energy dense meal requires massive amounts of physical activity to shed this excess energy.

High-intensity exercise
During high-intensity exercise fat cannot be delivered to exercising muscles quickly enough. Since oxygen is needed for fat to be released from the fat cell, and during high-intensity training oxygen is scarce, fat use is dramatically decreased. Fat is imprisoned in the fat cells. This, in turn, means that the process that burns fat is reduced resulting in the body using more energy from carbohydrate, which is in the form of glucose. This is clearly illustrated by a world-class female athlete when running a 400 metre race. Although she has enough fat on her body to be used for energy to keep her alive for many days without food, during the final 100 metres of the race she may slow down or struggle as she nears the finish line, since her body is running out of energy.

This is a clear example of how during high-intensity

activity fat just cannot be delivered quickly enough to exercising muscles. During this sort of training, fatigue is reached very quickly and we experience heaviness in the muscles of the arms and legs. This build-up of 'heaviness' results from lactic acid, or muscle-waste product. Lactic acid is produced when glucose is used for fuel building up in the blood and muscles, forcing your muscles to feel hot and jelly-like. This is one reason that this type of activity can only be undertaken for a maximum of 30 seconds.

When you stop, the body clears this lactic acid away, allowing you to commence exercise again. When your glucose stores run low, muscle fatigue will not allow you to continue at high intensities. This is despite having enough fat stores to walk for days. If you were to continue, the activity would drop to low intensity where fat can be used. This, however, can be dangerous, as a substantial glucose supply to the brain and nervous system is needed.

High-intensity training uses different types of muscle fibres (type 2) to those used in aerobic/low-intensity training. The benefits of high-intensity training include:

- increased strength of muscles and connective tissue
- increased coordination and range of movement
- increased amount of muscle fibres (and therefore fat-burning sites)
- you can exercise for longer without feeling heaviness in your legs
- better recovery after exercise

- increased bone density from weight training, especially in the elderly and women

Because high-intensity training leaves you 'more puffed' than moderate-intensity training, it is thought to burn more energy and hence help you to lose more weight. In a recent journal study (*Medicine & Science in Sports & Exercise*, 2002) this was tested for the first time. High- versus low-intensity exercise was tested, but ensuring the participants in the study expended the same amount of energy. The findings of the study clearly showed that high-intensity exercise results in a greater oxygen debt after exercise. In other words, the participants were more puffed after the high-intensity weight training, especially in the first 20 minutes, and then from 45 to 60 minutes. The study concluded however that although there were greater differences in oxygen debt after high-intensity training, these differences were not significant enough to provide superior weight loss over low-intensity training. In a further study, which compared high-intensity and moderate-intensity exercise, despite the high-intensity group having twice the oxygen debt (being twice as puffed, if you like), the differences in energy used during the recovery wasn't significantly different. In fact, the high-intensity group used 38 grams of carbohydrate and 12.3 grams of fat, whereas the low-intensity group used 28 grams of carbohydrate and 9.8 grams of fat in the hour after exercise (*Journal of the American Collage of Nutrition*, 1997).

Choosing the best exercise for you

So, it is shown here that all exercise is good for you. It is good for your heart, lungs, muscles and general fitness. But not all exercise is equal when it comes to the most effective way to lose weight. In *The Fat-Stripping Diet* we described how challenging it is to shift stubborn weight that may have accumulated over the years if you exercise but still eat a typical Western diet. This still holds today. If you are serious about losing weight permanently, you need to above all: 1. eat a low EDI diet; and 2. increase your incidental activity.

As you've seen here, other forms of activity will increase the amount of energy you burn, so by all means get out and walk, swim, cycle, but for the best results you need to do these in conjunction with The Bilsborough Program.

One of the most disheartening things we see in the fitness industry is a person who trains for 20 weeks, whether it be in a gym or just walking their dog, yet doesn't get their desired results. Of course it's equally sad seeing a person get great results too quickly, which we know are just not sustainable, and then go back to their starting weight as their body rebels against this too-sudden, drastic change. A 1999 journal article from the *American Journal of Clinical Nutrition*, called the HERITAGE Family Study, showed that when men and women (nearly 600 in total) underwent fitness training without any intervention in their daily eating, weight loss was marginal. Subjects cycled for 30 minutes three times a week for 14 weeks and then for 50 minutes three times a week for 6 weeks, yet their body weight decreased only between 0.1 to

0.4 kilograms. These results are very demotivating, particularly if you really are making an effort to exercise.

The study clearly illustrates the challenges that Chelsea and Charles faced when trying to exercise to burn up all the energy they had eaten the night before. If the energy density of our meals is high (i.e. we eat whatever we feel like), we won't get the results we want, even if we exercise.

It is very important, when choosing an exercise program for yourself, to assess your own level of fitness. For the majority of people (the 60 to 65 per cent of the Western population who are overweight and don't go to the gym), a low energy density diet and aerobic training (such as walking or cycling) will have more advantages than a program of general dieting and weight training. The practical reasons are that an activity such as walking can be sustained for longer periods of time, usually longer than a weight-training session. For gym beginners, three sessions a week for one hour each is usually all they can manage. Walking may last for one to two hours at a time and be sustained for three to four times a week, sometimes even more. Other benefits of walking are that you can interact with a friend, partner, or children. For some people going to a gym, purchasing a home gym, and doing high-intensity exercise is simply not practical. If this is you, then your program, which of course should incorporate the Bilsborough Program, should consist of aerobic training. Don't underestimate the energy-burning properties of your legs and a good walk.

If you are a gym-goer, or interested in joining a gym, then

there are advantages. The key to a successful gym program, however, is to get out of the incorrect mindset that three one-hour sessions a week is all you need. You still will need a large backdrop of daily incidental activity too. If you are lucky enough to have a personal trainer, don't rely on him or her to perform miracles in the three hours you are in contact.

Combining aerobic training (such as walking, cycling or jogging) with weight training has been shown to provide further benefits in both fat loss and weight loss than either activity done alone. By combining these two types of exercise you build more muscle, and muscles burn fat. Second, walking at a good pace over an extended period releases a massive amount of fat to be used. You then have the useful combination of plenty of fat being released into your bloodstream and plenty of muscle to burn this fat. Some studies have shown that in a period of about 20 weeks you can lose in the vicinity of 16 kilograms this way.

We are frequently asked to recommend the best exercise-training program. Combination training (i.e. moderate-intensity walking *and* weight training) has been shown to be extremely effective not only in burning massive amounts of energy but, when combined with a diet low in energy density, in promoting weight and fat loss. Of course if you cannot get to a gym, then some hand weights used at can be home very effective. It is important, however, to incorporate the Bilsborough Program into your training. As we have continuously stressed, there is no point exercising three times a week if you are totally inactive for the rest of the time (165 hours).

Exercise scientists love to debate whether high-intensity is better than low-intensity exercise for weight loss. We have shown you that there is no specific right answer. *The best program is the one that can be sustained for the longest period of time.* For some this may be walking, while for others it may be the gym. If you're a highly trained athlete, then your training will be vastly different from that of a mum with four children who has never exercised before. For very fit people high-intensity training has definite advantages over moderate-intensity training, but how many of you reading this book are highly trained athletes? If you have trained regularly all your life, then the amount of fat and glucose that your body uses will be different from that of a chubby person who has at best walked on and off for years. Finally, if you can't be physically active through structured exercise, be very active through incidental activity.

Don't forget your health

Although we have categorically stated that exercising three times a week *may not* have the precise benefits we want for weight loss, as our backdrop of incidental activity each day may be too low, there are many other benefits to cycling or walking three times a week. In a 1999 article in the *American Journal of Clinical Nutrition*, it was found that fit, overweight men had a better chance of avoiding heart disease (such as stroke and heart attack) than a lean unfit man! In fact as little as two hours of vigorous physical activity per week was shown to reduce the risk of cardiovascular disease by a factor of five.

This clearly shows that although weight is important for good health, fitness is essential for perfect health. Many unfit, lean men and women naively believe that, because they don't have excess flab, they don't have to exercise.

Although a total review of all exercise programs and weight loss programs is impossible in this book, we have attempted to summarise as many studies as possible. Over a 20 week period exercising three to four times a week and eating a typical diet that is high in energy density may result in just a 2 kilogram weight loss, which is a poor weight-loss result. Whereas a low energy-dense diet can result in a minimum of 7 kilograms of weight loss. At B Personal we have followed the progress of people on a low energy density diet in a 20 week period and seen over 10 kilograms being lost. Following a low energy density diet combined with some weight training can also provide some sensational results, as resistance training builds lean muscle and muscle is where you burn fat. The more muscle you have, the more fat you can burn. As we get older we lose muscle mass so resistance training, especially for elderly people, can be a great way to lose weight.

Exercise and the Energy Diet – putting it all together

The exercise sessions described above clearly show that what we consider to be a good workout can in reality have little effect on burning the vast volumes of energy we eat. This is one of the key reasons that we devised the Bilsborough

Program, so that incidental activity can provide a springboard for all other physical activity.

In a recent study, two groups of normal-weight men were fed either a daily diet of 11 600 kJ (to simulate a typical Western man's diet) or a diet of 14 000 kJ (to represent what a man who overeats consumes).

If we consider that Charles consumed upwards of 18 000 kJ in one day, we could probably assume that the 14 000 kJ group typify a weekday of bad eating. Half the men from each group did some activity (cycling for 40 minutes three times a week). The other half did no activity at all. The study then measured exactly what energy was metabolised by their bodies and what energy was left over at the end of the day. The energy balance graph is shown below and reinforces the theme of the book: you cannot lose weight if you eat more energy than you burn up.

THE ENERGY DIET WITH AND WITHOUT EXERCISE

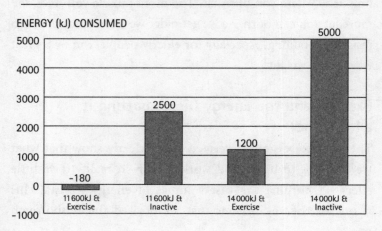

ENERGY (kJ) CONSUMED

Men who consume a typical Western diet (11 600 kJ), which is high in animal fat and low in fibre, and are not physically active have a surplus or leftover daily energy of about 2500 kJ. Naturally, this will be stored as fat. Men who follow a typical Western diet but manage to do some physical activity burn off more energy than they consume, but only if they are keeping their energy in balance. They have burnt off only a fraction more than their intake – 180 kJ, or the energy contained in an apple. Men who ate a 14 000 kJ diet (which probably reflects most men out there) and got some exercise used about 2600 kJ of energy. Even with exercise they still had about 1200 kJ left over energy from their day's eating. Eating an extra 2200 kJ a day will certainly not lead to any weight loss. For the men who ate 14 000 kJ and were inactive, they had a 5000 kJ of energy left over per day. For big eaters who are inactive, 5000 kJ extra kilojoules a day is grossly above human energy requirements and typifies a common trait in twenty-first-century Western society: passive gluttony.

A question that you may ask is in what form is this energy stored, fats or carbohydrates? Interestingly enough, the group who ate 14 000 kJ and were inactive and stored over 5000 kJ, stored 4100 of those kJ from fat (or 108grams, or 81 per cent). The group that ate 11 600 kJ and were inactive stored 2500 kJ of which 1000 kJ (26 grams) came from fat and 1300 kJ (77 grams) came from carbohydrate. This 77g of carbohydrate is stored in the human body as glycogen, not fat. We still get frustrated when people say that carbohydrates get stored as fat. Carbohydrates are never stored as fat. They are stored as glycogen in either the liver or muscle.

Working extensively in the fitness industry in Australia, we have a chance to observe people's perception about being active. Keep asking yourself the question 'Does doing physical activity three times a week for an hour classify someone as being an active person?' As you can see over and over again this amount of activity may not be enough to shift the large loads of energy that we eat. On the other hand, if you control your energy intake and follow the Bilsborough Program, then three one-hour sessions may be quite beneficial.

The key to achieving your goals

One of the keys to a successful exercise program is to create a supportive environment for yourself, and hence your exercise program. A supportive environment means that whether you are at home, at work, or actually participating in your physical activity, everything and everyone provides a positive reinforcement of your program. Creating a supportive environment can be the key then to achieving your goals.

Spend some time planning your program, just as an athlete spends time planning. Although exercise can be spontaneous, it is better adhered to when planned, and when children are involved this is even more crucial. Planning can include contacting a training partner, looking for volunteers from the family who will sacrifice one morning a week for a walk, wording up family on your exercise plans, planning times that you know you can keep. (There's no point saying to yourself that you will get up at 5.30 a.m. on a day you have to work for 15 hours.) Remember too to organise cooking menus and set aside time for yourself.

The concept of a training partner, such as someone who you go to the gym with or someone you walk with, is very important to the success of your supportive environment. When choosing a training partner and times to train, it may be beneficial to schedule your training partner at the end of the week, when you are more likely to be unmotivated and hence more inclined to skip your session. Many people exercise early on in the week but tend not to do so late in the week. If you have exercised very well during the week and then come Friday it's wet, you may be inclined to stay indoors, whereas your training partner will push you to simply rug up and train. Scheduling an early Friday morning walk that lasts for 90 minutes before work for example is a very challenging task as by this time you will undoubtedly be tired. If your training partner understands this then you are both working towards this challenge and you are more likely to succeed together.

When finding your training partner, remember that your goals may be different to theirs. Your motivation to start a program may be greater than your partner's, so don't initiate a five-morning-a-week program with your partner because your motivation should at least get you through two sessions on your own. Suggesting a five-day-a-week training program with your exercise partner can come unstuck if your partner misses two sessions, loses motivation, begins to feel negative or likely to fail. Do all you can to keep the environment supportive. Family members make the best training partners because they are more likely to understand your goals, plus there is the convenience of proximity.

Summary

The human body was designed to be active. In the context of human evolution, exercising three times a week for an hour would be considered to be a small amount of physical activity. After all, it accounts for only 2 per cent of our week. It means for the remaining 98 per cent of the week we are essentially inactive. This is why we have devised the very simple and easy to use Bilsborough Program. You can increase your daily energy expenditure by over 200 per cent, without any fuss. Low energy dense meals coupled with daily physical activity, both incidental and structured, will bring about the weight loss changes you are looking for. If you're serious and committed, then you too can achieve these goals.

CONCLUSION

Everywhere you look it seems there is something that reminds us of food, from adverts on television telling us about the newest 'meal deal' to magazines showing mouth-watering dishes. Even walking through a shopping mall, we are bombarded with sweet aromas of freshly baked goods.

Why is it that some people can eat and eat and eat, yet stay wafer-thin, while others diet and exercise, only to lose faith in both when they fail to deliver the desired weight decrease? Genetics do admittedly play a part, but let's not use that as an excuse to give up. Changing our eating behaviour and ensuring real food education in this food-saturated environment are the two most significant keys to winning through to permanent weight loss.

Eating behaviour and the successful dieter

The interaction between eating behaviour and weight loss is extremely significant. Actually, it's more accurately 'human' behaviour that we need to consider.

People who are successful at losing weight don't have to hide food, live in denial, or yo-yo their weight. Studies show that people who have been successful at losing weight and keeping it off have certain characteristics. And chief among them is patience.

HAVE YOU THE TRAITS OF A SUCCESSFUL DIETER?

	YES	NO
Sincere intent		
Positive body image		
Confidence		
Self-control		
Discipline		
Motivation		
High self-esteem		
Educated in the area of concern		
High level of self-efficacy		
Patience		

For the serial dieter, addressing some of these issues first may be the key to successful weight loss. Ticking yes to the majority of boxes suggests you are halfway there.

There is no finish line

When it comes to changing one's mindset to achieve successful and permanent weight loss, the greatest change is to acknowledge that there is no finish line. This means that any results that you get during an eight-week period can disappear if you believe that you can revert back to your original diet and lifestyle. Unfortunately, many people successfully lose weight, look great for a while but then slip back to the restaurant food, wine, sleeping in instead of being active, and eating plenty of energy from large food portion sizes. The motivation seems to have vanished and the weight creeps back on. Remember that keeping weight off is as challenging as losing weight in the first place.

With this book, you should be able to apply the key concept to all your grocery shopping, cooking, dining out and exercise. By doing this you make the transition from a diet to a lifestyle. Your lifestyle then allows you to eat low energy dense foods and get regular exercise. Success with any program will depend on how much the program becomes integrated with your life. The greater the integration, the more likely you will get both short-term and long-term weight loss. If walking or exercising three times a week is going to be a part of a one-off eight-week program, and that's it, your program is doomed to failure. If your eating is structured for only twelve weeks, then by the sixteenth week you will be right back where you started from.

Sticking to the plan

There is more to weight loss than simply following an eating plan, as most people struggle to follow even a seven-day eating plan without cheating. Other factors such as developing a supportive environment is essential. Being honest with yourself is also a key ingredient to successful weight loss, and viewing yourself in a positive way will enhance self-esteem and confidence and spur you on to achieving even better weight loss.

The road to success, or some healthy advice . . .

- Manipulate the environment so that it doesn't manipulate you.
- Shop at the supermarket more, eat out less.
- Plan ahead – make a shopping list.
- Find foods you enjoy and learn to make a healthy version of it.
- Eat foods in a simpler format – so you know what's in them!
- Take food to work.
- Eat healthy snacks.
- Eat in only one room.
- Eat only at scheduled times.
- Keep food records – you'll be amazed at how much you eat.
- Eat from home as often as possible.
- Avoid eating every time you sit in front of the TV.
- Try to discover why you eat. Do you eat because you're

hungry or because you happen to walk past a fast food outlet and it smells inviting?

- Find out what emotions cause you to eat certain foods.
- Do you eat because you are depressed or to soothe or to reward yourself?
- Make small changes, one by one. Don't take on 50 changes at once.
- Remember, change always demands an adjustment period. Along the way expect teething problems. Confront them, deal with them, learn from them, and continue forward.
- Don't expect miracles. Be realistic about your weight loss or you will be left despondent when you haven't achieved goals that were unobtainable.
- Address your health through diet and exercise and *then* focus on weight loss.
- Don't set a figure on your weight reduction on Day 1 (e.g. 'I want to lose 20 kg by Christmas'). Just start focusing on the small changes you can make now.
- Don't make excuses or reasons for why you didn't exercise. If you set out to achieve a task, complete it.
- Combine any dieting program with exercise – this is a MUST!

INDEX

Also from Penguin Books

The Fat-Stripping Diet
Shane Bilsborough

Why can't you get rid of that tummy – even though the rest of your body is trim? Why don't you have defined abs and a taut bottom – even though you exercise?

These are common problems faced by men and women who lead busy, active lives. But now, help is at hand. *The Fat-Stripping Diet* means you get the body shape you want by losing fat, not muscle. Shane Bilsborough shows you how to achieve an energising diet – and the good news is that carbohydrates are back!

With lots of motivating tips and the latest scientific research, this diet is not just a weight-loss program but the first step to a longer, healthier life.

7 Days to Strip Fat Forever
Shane Bilsborough

The Fat-Stripping Diet took Australia by storm with its no-nonsense advice on fat loss.

Now Shane Bilsborough takes you one step closer to perfect health and fitness. The secret to losing weight is to have small meals often, and with his '7 meals a day for 7 days', Shane shows you how easy it is.

You will discover:
- 7 successful strategies to lose weight
- easy eating plans to help you take control
- the 7x7 Fat-Reducing Plan – a complete eating program
- the 7x6 Heart Plan – for healthy hearts and bodies
- how to eat just enough food
- how much exercise will work off your last meal
- inspiring 'before and after' case studies

On these flexible eating plans, you can eat carbohydrates, you can eat protein, you can even eat chocolate. Losing fat is not just about how much you eat but how you eat it, and some simple tricks will show you ways to reduce your fat intake and reduce your body fat – forever.

Living Lite
Sandy Frazer

In 1992, I was 30 kilograms overweight. By 'Living Lite', I lost it and have successfully maintained my ideal weight ever since.

Living Lite contains over 120 original recipes that include creamy pasta sauces, chocolate cakes and many other 'forbidden' foods.

Clever substitutions allow you to eat healthily and guilt-free. I devised these recipes to trim down but more importantly to stay trim. Now I share them with you.

Sandy Frazer

Inside you will find:
- Innovative and easy recipes that can help you lose and control weight
- Tasty dishes that eliminate fat but not flavour
- Shopping guides, eating ideas & food preparation hints for cutting down on fat and calories

See how easy and delicious low-fat cooking can be, with recipes for goodies such as crumbed crab cakes, lite laksa, cheesecake, chocolate pudding and many more.

This book is all you need for *LIVING LITE* every day!

Lite for Life!
Sandy Frazer

Sandy Frazer's first book on losing weight and healthy eating, *Living Lite*, has sold over 25000 copies, becoming an Australian number-one bestseller.

This all-new book provides over 150 low-fat and ultra-low-fat recipes for delicious dishes such as chicken nuggets and spicy fries, lime lentils with couscous, and chocolate mud cake. They're so good you won't believe they're low fat!

With ideas for breakfast, lunch and dinner, healthy 'junk' food, chocolate recipes and a seven-day menu plan, *Lite for Life!* gives you all you need to enjoy fantastic, guilt-free food.